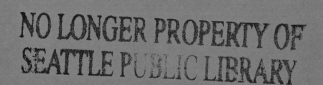

The WRINKLIES'™ GUIDE TO

Keeping Supple

New pursuits for old hands

Vicky Hales-Dutton

PRION

First published in Great Britain in 2012

Prion Books
an imprint of the
Carlton Publishing Group
20 Mortimer Street
London W1T 3JW

Illustrations: Peter Liddiard
Text: Guy Croton

A catalogue record of this book is available from the British Library.

ISBN: 978 1 85375 838 6

Printed in the UK by CPI Group (UK) Ltd, Croydon, CR0 4YY

10 9 8 7 6 5 4 3 2 1

CONTENTS

FOREWORD

I have this rule, had it for years, that I never discuss health or aches and pains with anyone younger than myself. It would only bore them, or disgust them, as it did me when I was young and heard oldies grinding on about their backs, their knees, their water works, their operations. "What do you expect, at your age," I can hear them thinking, for the young move their lips when thinking.

So if asked today by persons of a younger persuasion, I say "Fine, fine," and change the subject. If I get caught limping or staggering or even worse falling, I say "Glad you noticed, good trick, eh, I used to work in a circus, the old magic is still there."

However, if I am with someone of my generation, then certainly I will grind on about the state of play, body wise, knowing he or she is just waiting for a break in the flow and then they will jump in and tell me blow-by-blow the latest on their dodgy back, knackered knee, new ticker.

Just had lunch with one dear old friend from Cumbria – Lord Bragg of Wigton, a fine figure of a man – and I told him I had strained my back doing something stupid, God knows what, and was in agony, could hardly walk, sleep and certainly not swim. I don't take pain killers, have never found physiotherapy to work, so that's it, I moaned, it will take three weeks of being sensible before it gets better.

He immediately told me how he had done the same thing, and was equally in agony, but he had found great relief with Voltarol Heat Patches. So I rushed out and bought a packet, not cheap, and do you know, in two days the relief was amazing. Not quite playing football again, but back to normal physical, supple, healthy, energetic elderly life. For there is such a thing, oh yes, for we folks over 60. Ok then, 70 in my case. Steady on.

I don't hold with any gym work, press ups and weights and all that stuff, sounds awfully dangerous and a bit unseemly if there are other people watching. And I don't do any running. But then I never did.

Walking though, that is brilliant, for anyone of any age. You know, one foot in front of the other, simple really, no need for diagrams and certainly no need for any gear like heavy-duty walking boots.

Swimming, that is my other major way of keeping lovely and supple. I go three times a week, either to Cockermouth Baths when we are in Lakeland or Kentish Town Baths in London. The point about swimming is that you are not pounding any joints, hammering any muscles. The water takes the strain, takes the weight, but you are still exercising the old arms and legs, tums and bums and other bits too personal too mention, the sort of intimate details and descriptions I save for my elderly friends.

Hunter Davies

INTRODUCTION

Welcome to *The Wrinklies' Guide to Keeping Supple!*
Having just picked up – possibly even purchased, with
any luck – a book with the word "wrinklies" on the cover,
chances are that you are one of us. You are a *wrinkly*!
You've lived long enough to know that it doesn't really
matter if your trousers are tucked in your socks or your
hair has gone a little astray. You've managed to open the
front cover and thumb your way to page six, so there's not
much wrong with your hands, but what about the rest of
you? Are you shaping up or seizing up? Are you ready to
take on the next challenge in this fast-moving world? First
though, there are a few things to discuss.

Keeping supple?

Helping you to get back into shape is what this little book
is all about. Our aim is to make your muscles stronger,
your sinews sing again and get your joints to jump and
jangle. Keeping supple is not as hard as you might think,
and is certainly not the sole preserve of those young
enough to wear lycra. It just requires a little effort and a
positive attitude. So, once you have read this book, you
will have taken your first step towards becoming fitter,
healthier and more flexible.

What's it all about?

Do you remember "Let's Get Physical", the top ten hit for
the lovely Olivia Newton-John back in 1981? In her music

video she donned a towelling headband together with the ubiquitous hot pink lycra, and urged us all to:

Let's get physical, physical
I wanna get physical
Let's get into physical
Let me hear your body talk, your body talk
Let me hear your body talk

Both the song and the video offered some light relief from the craze for Jane Fonda's workouts and a humorous face to the business of worshipping the body beautiful. However, we know that the gym is not for everyone and we all need to choose the exercise that works for us.

Exercise for wrinklies

We begin with a detailed chapter on stretching to set the pace and get you up and moving. Stretching is a recurring theme and is essential for everyone who wishes to remain fit and supple – when in doubt, stretch, stretch, stretch! Chapters then follow on walking, swimming, cycling and yoga.

Perhaps you thought you would never need any advice about walking – after all, you've been doing it for quite a few decades without any problems – but you might be surprised. It's a great form of exercise at any age, but there's plenty you need to know if you want to make the most of it and keep yourself lean and limber.

The same goes for swimming. The thought of a cold pool might send you spinning for the kettle and a nice cup of tea, but with our sensible, down-to-earth tips and advice maybe you will decide to take the plunge, as swimming is one of the very best low-impact forms of exercise for keeping your muscles, joints and bones healthy.

Cycling is slightly more adventurous but it's a wonderful form of exercise that will get you out and about, while also providing an invigorating surge of fresh air, adrenalin and sheer feel-good health and fitness.

Yoga is the most contemplative of all exercises. This book offers a wide range of exercises for the more flexible among you, with detailed instructions on how to adopt the poses and a sprinkling of diagrams to help you.

Other ways to stay supple

As if all that isn't enough, we provide a closing chapter of other exercises that are ideal for those of greater vintage. From the enigmatic mysteries of "core stability" (not something involving nuclear reactors, but actually exercises for a stronger torso and better posture), we take you through a detailed all-over body workout, with dedicated routines for a stronger back, a flat stomach, supple arms and gorgeously toned legs. There is even lots of information on the concept of "warming down" (which used to be known as "cooling off") to make sure your exercise leaves you feeling relaxed and energized.

Meat and drink

Keeping supple isn't just about exercise, of course – it's about laying off the pork pies and avoiding those unwanted extra pounds, as well. What you eat and drink is important at any stage in your life, but when you get to our age, you essentially have a choice: you can either ignore all the good advice out there and eat or drink to your heart's content but risk the consequences; or you can say "Let's get physical" and start (or continue) eating for your continued health and physical contentment. Suffice to say that the latter is always the best way. Our chapter on diet for suppleness provides lists of all the best – and worst – foods to eat in later life, both for general health and increased suppleness. It's not all gloom and doom, either – there is information about what you might think of as forbidden fruit or naughty tidbits that are actually very good for our health and well-being, such as red wine (in moderation!) and dark chocolate (likewise).

Joint care

Finally, and with a view to any aches and pains you might develop as you start a new exercise programme, we take a detailed look at how to look after your joints. There is lots of good advice about dietary supplements and hot and cold treatments.

If you come through the latter stages of our jaunt through superannuated suppleness without any hitches, you could always turn to the table of Daily Suppleness Challenges at the very back of the book. These combine some of all of the above forms of exercise in imaginative ways and are designed to test even the fittest readers.

So, to quote Miss Newton-John one last time, "Let me hear your body talk", and here's to keeping supple.

Chapter 1

WHY KEEP SUPPLE?

Do you remember when you felt physically invincible?
When you could go anywhere, do anything, fall over,
get up, jump as high as you liked and stay up all night
without getting tired? At all? Perhaps that was a long time
ago, or maybe – if you're lucky – it was yesterday! Well,
chances are that apart from the wonderful care-freedom
and boundless energy of youth that drove you along so
compellingly, part of what you made you feel like that was
… suppleness.

What is Suppleness?

At its most technical, suppleness "… is demonstrated in
the wide range of movement that is possible in a joint or at
joint complexes". If that sounds complicated, suppleness
is similar to flexibility. The definition of flexibility and/
or suppleness is that your muscles, bones and joints work

together to produce the maximum range of movement without pain or injury.

Suppleness affects bodily movement and posture. It contributes to fitness by determining the range limits through which limbs can or cannot move. Its presence or absence will very much influence a person's potential ability in a sport skill that requires a high degree of bodily flexibility, such as hurdling or gymnastics. In a nutshell, it is what allows you the kind of movement that as a youngster you probably took for granted – but perhaps not anymore ...!

In everyday life, the presence of suppleness in your body helps you to avoid injuries when you are confronted by the need for sudden bodily twists or distortion, such as when you are doing awkward jobs around the house or garden – like washing the dog or trimming a hedge – or getting into and out of a small, cramped car.

Though it is perfectly possible to possess both stamina and strength in a body that is stiff and inflexible, the attainment and maintenance of suppleness is an important aspect of fitness and body efficiency – at any age. It does not matter how strong you are; if your muscles and joints are not sufficiently supple you will not be able to bring that strength to bear in a practical and sustainable form.

Although most exercise promotes muscle suppleness, as we demonstrate throughout this book, it should be noted that some forms of exercise can actually lead to muscle shortening. This is particularly the case as you get older.

Therefore, after exercise it is always important to "warm down" (or "cool down", if you prefer) with a series of gentle stretching exercises. There is plenty of advice on this throughout the book, together with detailed information about "warming up", which should be undertaken prior to any form of exercise, and which helps the muscles and joints make ready for the extra suppleness that the exercise in question should foster.

When Muscles, Bones and Joints Begin to Age ...

Like waves crashing endlessly on a shore, the years roll by inexorably. Nobody can avoid the passage of time – unless they die young and pretty – which most of us try to avoid. There are the usual tell-tale signs: your eyes stop working properly; your teeth fall out; your hair goes grey (or falls out as well); people stop looking at you (in fact, you become invisible!); the cat no longer recognizes you; and your bones and joints begin to ache.

Why do they do this? Well, it's because they are becoming less supple. It's an unavoidable part of ageing and a "joint" thing in more ways than one. Our muscles, joints and bones are all so inextricably linked together that one cannot really operate at all without the others. And the triple whammy is that, as you age your muscles lose mass, your bones lose density and your joints stiffen up. This usually starts to happen as you enter roughly the fifth decade of your life. Life is unkind in three ways simultaneously, if you like – but the good news is that you can do something about it.

Avoiding Osteoporosis

That "something about it" is of course exercise, the pursuit of which is presumably what inspired you to buy this book, which of course is aimed at those of us who wish to remain supple. Exercise will increase your muscle mass once more, will help your joints to become more fluid and work better and, perhaps most importantly of all as you enter your twilight years, will improve the density of your bones. This will help you to avoid the spectre of osteoporosis – a very serious spectre at that, with a particularly dark and foreboding habit, cowl and scythe ...

Osteoporosis (meaning "porous bones" in ancient Greek) is a bone disease that can lead to the increased risk of fracture. It particularly afflicts older people, for the reasons given above. Post-menopausal women are also especially vulnerable.

Although it has no obvious symptoms, osteoporosis makes its presence felt among older people through the greater incidence of falls that they tend to experience. (Yes, it's depressing to note that another symptom of ageing is that you are prone to falling over rather a lot – whether you had that "last" whisky or not.) The increased risk of falling associated with ageing leads to fractures of the wrist, spine and hip, all of which are weakened by the onset of osteoporosis. The risk of falling, in turn, is increased by impaired eyesight due to any cause (for example, glaucoma), as well as lots of other charming age-related conditions such as balance and movement disorders (for example, Parkinson's disease) and dementia. So it's a vicious circle. However, with its anabolic effect (meaning it affects the metabolism), exercise can not only slow and diminish the creeping nature of osteoporosis, but increase overall strength and fitness to reduce the likelihood of the falls that accompany it. (That's the science bit over with!)

The Importance of Healthy Muscles

So, healthy bones are the best old bones – but they aren't much use unless they are accompanied by toned, flexible muscles. Again, this is where exercise is the key. It's never too late to build up muscles and make them strong again. Weight training, physiotherapy, gardening, walking – any form of activity, really – will all make your muscles work harder and perform better. Try any form of exercise covered in this book and we guarantee that your muscles will benefit. And the greater strength and suppleness of those muscles will mean that your joints and bones will improve a little every time you move, as well.

However, exercise is not the only factor in maintaining healthy muscles, at any time of life. Lifestyle and diet also play a huge part and it is particularly important not to neglect these as you embark on a course of exercise. Think of the three things as a sort of Holy Trinity for a better, longer and more pain-free life: exercise; diet; healthy lifestyle. Believe it or not, this magic formula applies as much now as it ever did earlier in your life.

KEEP YOUR MUSCLES HEALTHY WITH PROPER NUTRITION

1 Eat a balanced diet as outlined on pages 146–149.

2 Avoid refined grains, such as white bread and white rice. Replace refined grains with wholegrains, such as wholegrain bread, oatmeal and brown rice. Wholegrain foods contain fibre, an essential part of growing and repairing muscles.

3 Eat plenty of fruit and vegetables. Fruit and vegetables are full of vitamins and minerals, including iron, calcium and vitamin D. These nutrients are vital to muscle health, whatever age you are.

4 Avoid eating more than the recommended amount of fruit, as it contains fructose. Fructose is a carbohydrate, which is a fuel your body needs during exercise. An excess of fructose, however, will lead to fat build-up.

5 Select low-fat or non-fat dairy products, like milk, cheese and yogurt. Dairy products are rich in calcium and aid in healthy bones. Strong bones are the foundation for building healthy muscles.

6 Get your protein from meat, poultry, fish, nuts, eggs and beans. Proteins are the building blocks for bones and muscles. Meat and poultry also contain iron, which is essential for healthy oxygenated blood.

KEEP YOUR MUSCLES HEALTHY WITH EXERCISE

1 Stretch before any type of exercise. Stretching warms up your muscles and increases flexibility. Stretching also reduces the risk of muscle pulls and other injuries.

2 Warm up before any rigorous activity. Warming up activates your muscles and slowly increases your heart rate. This reduces the shock on your body when playing an aggressive sport or performing an intense workout session.

3 Do exercises that increase your heart rate. Try a variety of cardiovascular activities to keep your heart active and healthy. Running, walking, swimming and cycling all provide cardiovascular workouts.

4 Vary your exercises often. Once your muscles become used to a routine, its effectiveness decreases dramatically.

5 Work all of your muscle groups in different combinations. For example, do a chest press on a balance ball instead of a bench. Not only will you work your chest muscles, but you will also work your hip and gluteus muscles.

6 Cool down after exercise to bring your heart down to its resting rate and to avoid muscle cramping.

Happy Joints

If your bones are in good shape and your muscles are pulling everything together like Popeye, the chances are that your joints will be doing well as well. But there are other things you can do to keep them happy.

The first and most obvious thing is to keep a close eye on your weight. While some of us become interestingly wasted and gaunt as we get older, many of us go exactly the opposite way and become, well, too heavy for our own good. If this is you, take steps to lose weight now!

The fact that you are reading this book is a good starting point, and the very process of trying to become more fit and flexible should mean that you lose weight automatically anyway. However, the simple fact is that if you are consuming more calories than you are burning, you will continue to pile on the pounds, whatever exercise you might be taking. This is what is known as your "caloric balance". Put basically, consume more calories than you burn and you put on weight, consume fewer than you burn and you lose weight. As that irritating meerkat on the television commercial would say, "Simples!".

"So, what's all this got to do with my joints?", you may ask. Well, the less weight your joints have to carry around, the less stress they will be under and the more efficiently and comfortably they will work. Get the pounds off and your joints will be happier.

Once again, a healthy diet can also benefit your joints. Foods high in calcium, such as milk, yogurt, broccoli, kale and figs are particularly helpful in this regard. Additionally, protecting your joints with knee and elbow pads during exercise or any other form of physical duress will help them keep you well into old age, as will the application of an ice pack whenever they get tired or sore.

Ageing Gracefully

One of the best things about keeping supple as you age is that you are less likely to turn into the bent old crone you are afraid you might become. Keeping your bones, joints and muscles in fine fettle will reap rewards in other directions, such as better posture and a generally more upright and lithe-looking stance. You will move better, too – more like Helen Mirren and less like Hilda Ogden. Or Pierce Brosnan instead of Stan Ogden.

In this regard, a strong bodily core is vital and a key component of remaining supple all over. Exercises designed specifically for a strong core – known in the trade as "core stability" – are a major component of Chapter 7, "Other Exercises for Keeping Supple". Perhaps you could try some of these before choosing a dedicated sport or devising your own exercise plan? Alternatively, have a stab at one of the "Daily Suppleness Challenges" on pages 173–176.

However you decide to go about keeping supple, do make the effort. Sometimes it might feel like really hard work – we all have off days, or days when exercise is the last thing that we feel like doing – and maybe walking the cat around the hearth rug might seem more appealing. However, keeping supple will pay dividends, no matter how old you are, how much you might think you have let yourself go, or whatever your conscience is telling you. Age supply and you will age gracefully – and isn't that a great way to age if you have to age at all? And that's always going to be better than the alternative ... Remember what the author Geoffrey Parfitt had to say about ageing:

"People say that age is just a state of mind. I say it's more about the state of your body."

So, go on, do yourself a favour – keep supple!

Chapter 2

STRETCHING

If you want to look and feel your best, making time every day to stretch can help you to achieve your goals. Why not try it with your spouse or a friend for a bit of a laugh? It will break up your usual routine and help get you both in the positive mood you will need to adopt for some of the other sports and exercises covered in this book. Not only will stretching work to counter the muscle-shortening effects of exercise and help you develop toned, lean limbs (oh yes!), but it will also make you more supple and flexible.

Stretch for Life

If you've never really put much thought into how stretching can benefit your health and your body, this book will help you realize what an important part of any health and fitness regime stretching really is. It's a mantra throughout this tome: stretch, stretch, stretch! All the sports and exercises dealt with in these pages require it as a form of warm-up at the very least and regular stretching will help to reduce the risk of injury to your joints, muscles and tendons when you do exercise. Additionally, it's a great way of relieving any soreness and tension you may feel after a gruelling workout – when you "warm down" or "cool down", as you prefer.

Some people find they reach a plateau with exercise, and many health and fitness trainers recommend stretching to help you get and maintain the body you really want – no matter how wrinkly you might already be.

Impress your friends!

Spending just a few minutes in the morning doing some of the stretches in this book will help you to develop the kind of body that makes others envious! Impress your friends with your new-found flexibility and shiny, twanging muscles! But, once you've started, make sure you keep it up. The longer you keep stretching, the better you will look and feel.

Stretching develops your muscles in a different way from cardio- or other weight-based exercise. So, if you already put the time and effort into keeping fit, you should really be dedicating a set amount of time each day to stretching. It's also a great way to stay in shape if sweating it out in a gym simply isn't your thing.

Toning and lengthening muscles

While most forms of exercise will help you to burn calories and fat while strengthening and defining the muscles, stretching helps to tone and lengthen them. The result is that you can actually appear slimmer, even if you haven't lost any weight (isn't that brilliant?). However, if you practise regularly, the toning effects of stretching can make it easier to shift stubborn pounds and give you a more streamlined silhouette overall. Maybe you'll even feel like getting your little old black dress or dinner suit out of the wardrobe ... You may even find that you look taller – and definitely less bent – because some of the stretches in this book will help you to develop a better posture.

Stretch to relax and detox

If you need any more convincing, you'll be pleased to learn that stretching also has great benefits for the mind. While it does require a degree of concentration, to make sure you're doing each stretch correctly and to the best of your ability, you'll soon realize how relaxing it can be. We don't claim that it will banish Alzheimer's, more's the pity, but stretching will keep you feeling mentally fresh and sharp for longer.

Since stretching is best done in silence or to slow and soothing music, it can be almost like meditating. Setting aside just a few minutes in the morning for the following routines will help to put you in a positive frame of mind for the day to come. As you become more familiar with the different stretches, you can combine the movements with deep breathing and positive visualizations, which will help you to clear your mind from clutter. Forget about the cat being sick on the carpet or Aunty Maud's forthcoming 90th birthday party – just stretch away to your heart's content and clear your mind in the process.

Stretching is also a great way to stimulate the lymphatic system, which in turn helps to cleanse your body of toxins and boost circulation. So, if you're in need of a healthy boost, this book is also an ideal way to kick-start a detox diet.

How fit do I need to be?

The good news is that you don't have to be super-fit to do any of the stretches featured in this book. They are all designed to provide the perfect starting-point for beginners or older people with an existing medical condition – such as asthma – which may make it hard to do more energetic forms of exercise.

Mix and match your stretches

All of the stretches featured in this book aim to stretch out your major muscle groups. Each exercise targets a different part of the body, so why not combine a variety of different stretches each day for maximum results?

Each stretch should last for approximately 30 seconds and it's easy to see how you can combine different stretches to create a five or ten-minute daily routine. It's realistic to hold most of the stretches for three sets of around ten seconds, with a brief pause between. As long as you do what you feel comfortable with and don't pause for more than a couple of seconds at a time during the routine, you'll be doing enough to make it effective. If you can't always find time to do the routine in the morning, you can do it in the evening before bedtime. The reason that we recommend doing it in the morning is because of the mind- and body-boosting benefits mentioned above. But, as long as you are doing it regularly – ideally every day – then you will see results.

Setting goals

While setting goals with a few groups of stretches over several days is a great starting point, you should really aim to keep doing the stretches every day – for the rest of your life! The effects of stretching are cumulative, so if you suddenly stop for any length of time, you will lose more or less all the flexibility you've worked so hard to develop. This is because muscles respond more easily to other forms of exercise, such as running or cycling, which make the muscles contract and shorten. Even everyday walking will have this effect on the muscles, so you can see how essential stretching is to keeping you lithe and limber.

Getting Started

A good way to start is to spend a quiet afternoon flicking through this chapter to help familiarize yourself with the various stretches on offer. Once you've changed into some comfortable, loose-fitting clothes, you should switch off the television or any telephones and put on some soothing music. Designate a space in your home that's large enough for you to extend your arms and legs without knocking anything over, shut out the dog and/or cat, and begin your routine.

You should always make sure you are nice and warm before you stretch, so take a brisk walk around your home or march on the spot for a few seconds to help get your muscles into gear. You should always do this general warm-up, especially if you've just jumped out of bed in the morning. But, rest assured, there is little risk of pulling any muscles while doing the stretches, as long as you stick with what you're comfortable doing.

The golden rules of stretching

One golden rule to consider while stretching is that you should try to do each one to the best of your ability, but you should never push yourself so far that you feel pain. You don't want to set yourself back just as soon as you have started, so don't be tempted to overdo it. All the stretches require you to hold them for a maximum of three sets of ten seconds. It can be tempting to "bounce" while in the stretch to try to get down even further, if you are reaching for the floor, for example. However, this can strain the muscles, so you should avoid this. All the stretches are "static", which means they should be performed while keeping perfectly still.

If, once you've got used to stretching, you feel that you could improve your performance, you can try to increase the stretch by slowly and gently moving further into position. If you ever develop a persistent pain as a result of doing the stretches, make sure you see your doctor for advice.

It probably sounds silly, but you must remember to breathe at all times when stretching – believe us, your

other half will thank you for it! Many people have a
tendency to hold their breath as they hold certain poses,
which isn't advisable. Make sure you breathe deeply
and slowly throughout the routine, because it will help
deliver oxygen to the muscles and make the stretches more
effective.

Don't give up!

Exercise is easy to let slip when you're feeling under the
weather, and it's fine to give your body a break every now
and then. However, if you ever feel like you want to give
up, read these top motivational tips:

- Visualize how you will look and feel if you stick to the
  programme rather than letting it slip.

- Remember that waking up a few minutes earlier to
  perform stretches will not encroach massively on your
  sleeping time. You'll feel much more alert from doing
  the stretches than you would for having the extra time
  in bed.

- Not only is stretching good for your body but it's good
  for your mind, too. So, even if you're feeling down, or
  just plain old and tired, it's the perfect thing to do!

What You Need

You don't need a great deal of equipment to do the
stretches in this chapter, although there are a few things
that may be worth purchasing. For starters, at the very
least you should get your hands on a few good pieces of

clothing that are comfortable, breathable and made from a nice, stretchy material so that they won't restrict your movements.

Equipment

The amount of equipment you acquire to help with your stretching is up to you – there are plenty of pieces of kit available that are designed to create an unstable base and make your core muscles work really hard. These range from wobble boards to medicine balls, exercise balls, resistance bands and even adjustable cable pulley machines if you're in the gym. However, these are all pretty hi-tech items and you might feel they are not for you. For the purposes of this book, at the most we recommend an exercise ball and/or a wobble board for variation. Hand weights and ankle weights can be used (but not if you're new to exercise or have back problems) – but make sure they are not too heavy. Small cushions or folded towels make ideal padding during exercises which involve lying on the floor or kneeling.

What to wear

When stretching, avoid wearing clothing that will restrict your movements and choose clothes in which you can exercise comfortably, such as a T-shirt and leggings, tracksuit bottoms or shorts. Cotton and natural fibres are cooler than man-made ones, and it's best to wear layers that you can remove as necessary, in case you get hot. Wear trainers or exercise in bare feet – don't work out in socks because they look silly and anyway you might slip. Remove jewellery and belts, and tie your hair back if it is long.

Where, When and How Much to Stretch

Stretching should be fun and stress-free. Remember, you are doing it to become more supple, not more tense, so find a quiet place to call your own for half an hour or so and clear your mind of as many distractions as you can before you start!

Where to stretch

Find a quiet, comfortable, clutter-free space to work out in. You need a non-slip surface such as an exercise mat or a carpet to protect your spine and prevent bruising. If possible, try to exercise in front of a full-length mirror so that you can check what you are doing. Don't worry – only you will be able to see yourself, unless your other half is along for the ride, of course!

When to exercise

You should wait at least an hour after eating before exercising, but otherwise you can perform the exercises in this chapter at any time of the day. Choose the time that suits you best, whether it's a morning session to give you a burst of energy at the start of the day or an evening one to help you unwind after a busy day. However, never exercise immediately before going to bed, because you'll find it difficult to get to sleep.

How many exercises?

When you are stretching, it's the quality of the movement that counts above all, so start gently and build up the number of repetitions as you become fitter and more

29

limber. Don't attempt to do too much too soon. In general you should aim for one set (usually six to eight repetitions) of each exercise before moving on to the next one.

Concentration and focus

To get the most benefit from each exercise, you need to concentrate on how and where you are moving. By doing this you are more likely to move correctly and safely. This will also help you to interpret the way your body responds to each move and judge more accurately the correct state of tension or relaxation that is required. Use positive thoughts while you are exercising and focus on what you are doing right. Telling yourself that you are doing well can make you do even better.

Breathing

Breathing is something we all do without thinking but it can be consciously controlled. Correct breathing comes from the deepest area of the lungs, but most of us take shallow, rapid breaths and use only the top third of the lungs. Breathing properly encourages effective oxygenation of the blood, allowing muscles and organs to work efficiently. It also relaxes muscles, releases tension and enables you to contract your inner unit properly. You need to practise abdominal, or diaphragmatic, breathing, which allows the lungs to fill and empty with minimal effort. This will make your exercising much more effective – though you will find it quite difficult to do at first. Here's how you do it:

1 Sit in a comfortable position with your back supported. Place one hand on your chest and the other on your

abdomen just below the breastbone. If the hand on your chest moves more than the one on your abdomen as you breathe, then your breathing is mainly in the upper chest. Try to breathe so that only your lower hand is moving.

2 Now place both hands on your abdomen just below the ribs. Breathe in slowly through your nose. Pause for a few seconds then breathe out through your mouth, letting out as much air as possible, feeling your abdomen fall as your diaphragm relaxes.

3 Repeat three or four times.

Right – now you should be all set to stretch! All you need now is a positive attitude ...

Stretching Exercises

Try these proven body-stretchers to really wake you up and get you on the move!

FULL BODY REACH-UP
This exercise opens and strengthens your shoulders, lengthens your spine and neck and improves your posture. Keep your arms straight throughout the exercise.

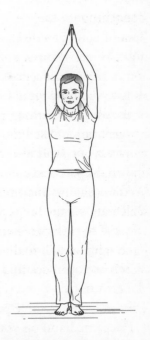

1 Stand with your feet close together, knees soft, spine in

neutral (normal) position (see standing pelvic tilt, page 34) and abdominal muscles contracted.

2 Slowly raise your arms, bringing your palms together above your head.

3 Take your arms back down to the starting position.

4 Perform four repetitions.

TORSO ROTATIONS

Gradually increase the range of movement as you do this exercise, reaching across your torso with your opposite hand as you do so. The twisting action should force you to come up onto the toes of your opposite foot.

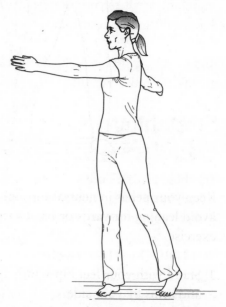

1 Keep your pelvis in neutral (normal position) and stand with your feet hip-width apart and knees slightly bent.

2 Rotate your torso to one side then the other, increasing the range of movement as you do so. You should feel a slight stretch across your back and shoulders.

3 Perform five to ten repetitions.

SIDE BENDS

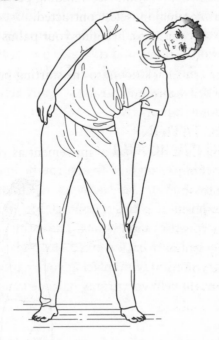

Keep your pelvis in neutral throughout and be careful to avoid leaning forwards or backwards while doing this exercise.

1 Stand with your feet hip-width apart, knees slightly bent and arms by your side.
2 Bend sideways at the waist and extend your left hand down your left leg, then stand up straight again.
3 Repeat on your right side. Bend a little further as you repeat the exercise, making sure you do not twist or bend your spine as you do so.
4 Perform five to ten repetitions.

CONTROLLING YOUR MOVEMENTS

Each movement should flow in a gentle, slow manner to let your muscles warm up and stretch naturally. Think about what you're doing and try to keep your body relaxed as you move. Never stretch further than is entirely comfortable or bounce into position. If any action hurts, you're not doing it properly.

STANDING PELVIC TILT

Pelvic tilting teaches you how to control the lumbar spine during exercise. The aim here is to practise finding your neutral spine position as this is essential for performing core stability exercises successfully. The action should be confined to your lower back – avoid any body sway. You may find that, to begin with, placing your hands either side of your waist will help you to stay balanced and correct any swaying.

1 Stand tall against a wall with your feet hip-width apart, arms by your sides.
2 Tilt your hips back and forth a few times – when tilting your pelvis forwards you should be able to fit your hand into the gap between your lower back and the wall as your lower back hollows. When you tilt your pelvis backwards you should feel your lower back press against your hand as it flattens. Aim to find the mid-range of this spinal movement, between the two extremes – this is your neutral spine position.

SPINAL CURL

This exercise will create flexibility and strength in your spine and relax your shoulders.

1 Stand with your feet hip-width apart and your knees "soft" (slightly bent). Bend your knees and put your hands on your thighs, just above the knees.
2 Push your buttocks away and let your lower spine curl downwards, making a concave shape.
3 Tightening your abdominal muscles, arch your lower back upwards, then release back to the concave shape.
4 Perform five to ten repetitions, increasing the movement with each repetition.

EASY CHEST STRETCH

This stretch targets the pectoral muscles, sometimes known as the "pecs", which are the major muscles at the front of the chest. It will also give your supraspinatus muscle, which runs along the top of your shoulder blades, a nice big stretch.

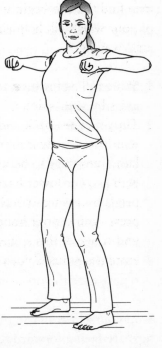

1 You can either stand with feet hip-width apart, or you can do this stretch while sitting on a chair. Whichever position you prefer, make sure that your back is straight and that your head and neck are in line with your spine.

2 Bring your arms up to shoulder level and bend from the elbows so that your hands are hovering in front of your chest. Make loose fists with your hands.

3 Leading from the elbow, gently rotate both arms backwards so that you're squeezing your shoulder blades together. Your chest will automatically push out a little.

4 Hold for ten seconds then release. Repeat this three times.

It's quite easy to get tired while doing this stretch but, if you persevere, you will get great results!

SHOULDER STRETCH

This is an easy stretch to do, and will really get your shoulders loosened up. It's great to do if you've been particularly stressed-out recently, because it will help to get rid of any built-up tension.

1 You can do this stretch from either a standing or a seated position.

2 Extend your right arm directly out in front of you so it's parallel with the floor.

3 Using your left hand, grip the back of your right arm between your elbow and your shoulder and use it to bring your right arm gently across the front of your chest. You should feel the stretch down the inner side of your right arm and across your right shoulder blade.

4 Hold the position for two sets of seven seconds and then repeat with the other arm.

Stop yourself from rotating round by making sure your hips are facing forwards at all times.

ARM STRETCH

This targets all the muscles in your upper arms – you'll be surprised at how easy it is to feel the stretch.

1 Stand in an open doorframe, with your abdominal muscles clenched tight and your body straight.
2 Hold on to the doorframe with your left hand just below shoulder level, or as high as is comfortable. Take a big step forwards so your left arm is extended out behind you. Keeping your hips facing forwards and your head and neck in line with your spine, rotate your upper body to the right until you feel the stretch in your left arm. Lean forwards to feel a greater stretch.
3 Hold for two sets of seven seconds then turn around, step forwards, and repeat with your right arm.

UPPER BACK STRETCH

Stretching out the muscles in the back will have a therapeutic effect on both body and mind. The back is one of the first areas to retain tension and stress, so stretching out the muscles will help to put you at ease and set you up for the day ahead.

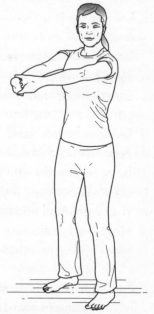

1 Stand with feet hip-width apart.
2 Interlink your fingers and push your hands out in front of you as far as possible. Your palms should be facing away from you.

3 Allow your upper back to relax by lowering your shoulders to their natural resting position.
4 Hold for ten seconds. You should feel the stretch between your shoulder blades. Pause for a brief moment, then repeat the stretch twice more.

If you find it hard to get your back to relax, just take a deep breath and lower your shoulders. This will have an instant relaxing effect.

MARCHING ON THE SPOT
This exercise increases hip and knee flexibility, strengthens hip flexor muscles, raises your pulse rate and body temperature and improves coordination between the right and left sides of your body.

1 Stand with your feet hip-width apart, your spine in neutral and your abdominal muscles braced to begin. Look straight ahead.
2 March on the spot for about a minute, lifting your knees as high as is comfortable and swinging each arm in turn towards your opposite knee as you march.

STANDING LEG LIFT
This exercise will help improve your balance, stabilize the pelvis and tone your thigh and hip muscles. Aim to keep your pelvis stable throughout.

1 Stand with your spine in neutral, feet slightly apart and arms by your sides.
2 Pull your navel in towards your spine and bring your left knee in towards your chest so that your big toe is

resting on the side of your right knee. Hold your knee with both hands, keeping your spine straight and your standing leg strong. You will need to drop your left hip down and lift the hip higher on the right side to keep your hips level at this point.

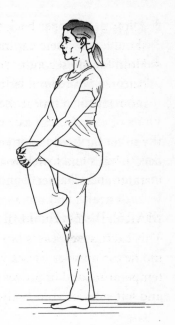

3 Hold for a count of three and then release.
4 Repeat with the other leg.
5 Perform four to six repetitions.

VARIATION

To make this exercise more difficult, after step 2 stretch your left leg straight out in front of you at hip height, holding on to the back of your thigh to support it. Release your arms and rest them on your buttocks, but keep your left leg extended in front of you. Hold for up to ten seconds and then lower your leg to the floor and repeat on the other leg. Perform four to six repetitions on each leg.

Conclusion

Remember, stretching is a useful complement to just about all forms of exercise – before and after – not least because it counters the effects of muscle-shortening that many kinds of exercise can cause. If you struggle with any of the other proposed sports or forms of exercise featured in this book, simply stick with the stretches featured in this chapter and Chapter 7 and you will still do your general level of health and fitness no end of good. If suppleness is the goal, then stretching performs the role ...

Chapter 3

WALKING FOR SUPPLENESS

Walking is probably something you have been doing all your life, but have you ever really considered it to be a form of exercise? Think about it: every time you crawl out of bed in the morning, what is the first thing that you do? Well, you walk! And when you crawl back into bed at night, you walk there, too. You wouldn't really get far without walking, would you – literally and metaphorically? But have you ever thought that this simple, automatic physical action could be just the thing to keep you nice and supple and in the prime of your later life?

The Benefits of Walking

There's no doubt about it, walking is good for you. It's good for your heart, it's good for your lungs, it's good for muscle and bone growth and strength maintenance and it's good for your feeling of wellbeing! Strong scientific evidence now supports the many benefits to health of regular walking.

"I have two doctors, my left leg and my right."
George Trevelyan, 1913

"Walking is the nearest activity to perfect exercise."
Professor J Morris and Dr Adrianne Hardman, 1997

THE HEALTH BENEFITS OF WALKING

- Walking is good for general health and longevity.
- Walking is good for increasing fitness.
- Walking is good for weight control.
- Walking is good for mental health.
- Walking is good for regaining health after illness.

Studies show that walking can:
- Reduce the risk of coronary heart disease and stroke.
- Lower blood pressure.
- Reduce high cholesterol and improve blood lipid profile.
- Reduce body fat.
- Enhance mental well-being.
- Increase bone density, hence helping to prevent osteoporosis.
- Reduce the risk of cancer of the colon.
- Reduce the risk of non-insulin-dependent diabetes.
- Help to control body weight.
- Help osteoarthritis.
- Help flexibility and co-ordination, hence reducing the risk of falls.

Whether you want to walk to improve your general health, to keep fit, to control your weight, or perhaps to recover from a period of ill-health, walking can help. It is something that can be done with grandchildren or older family members, it need cost you nothing, and it can fit in with any lifestyle, income bracket, culture or domestic circumstance.

Walking for General Health and Longevity

According to the British Medical Association and US Department of Health, regular participation in physical activity (such as walking) is associated with reduced mortality rates for both older and younger adults. In other words, walkers live longer!

In particular, walking has a high impact on cardiovascular disease. Fit and active individuals have around half the risk of cardiovascular disease compared to unfit, inactive people. This level of risk is similar to smoking, high blood pressure or high cholesterol in causing heart disease.

Fit older walkers are less likely to fall and suffer injuries such as hip fractures because their bones are strengthened; they are less likely to sustain injury because their joints have a better range of movement and their muscles are more flexible; they are less prone to depression and anxiety; they tend to be good sleepers; and they are better able to control body weight. Pretty compelling reasons to become a walker, *non*?

Warming Up for Walking

It might seem odd that you should have to "warm up" in order to walk, when it is something you have probably been doing all your life without thinking. However, the need for a warm-up all depends on your general physical state, how far you intend to walk, and just how quickly you mean to go.

A low intensity stroll at a 20-minute mile pace or slower does not require a warm-up. Simply start walking, find your comfort zone and continue. If a 20-minute mile pace is daunting for you, don't even think about such things! Just start pottering along at your own comfortable rate, safe in the knowledge that any walking is better than none, and that all walking is good exercise.

This is the great beauty of this form of exercise. You can do it at any time, any place and at your own pace. Of all forms of exercise, this is the one where you truly are the boss – completely in control. Go as fast or slow as you like, for just as far as you like, and it will do you good!

But what if you want to go a bit faster? Well then, as with any other form of exercise, it is a good idea to stretch out your walking muscles before starting. This is where flexibility comes in. Flexibility is the ability of the joints to move through their full range of motion, thus allowing muscles to approach their maximum stretch ability. Flexibility will vary from joint to joint and person to person. Don't be alarmed if you can't attain the same flexibility that your walking partner can. Simply work on getting the maximum flexibility possible for you. Older or not, an exercise-walker uses all the major muscle groups in the lower body; stretching these muscles and making sure the joints they influence are flexible, is important for a fluid, rhythmic walk.

Static stretching

The best kind of stretching for walking is called "static stretching". This simply means that you stretch the muscle slowly to its greatest possible length and hold it for about 10–30 seconds. Once you have done this, slowly release the tension on the muscle. Stretch until you feel a pulling sensation, with a slight bit of discomfort or a minor, dull ache. You should not feel pain, and above all you should not bounce or snap the muscle. Over time, stretching will produce a semi-permanent lengthening of the muscle; this will strengthen it and improve your walking. However, if you stop stretching, the muscle will soon shorten again, especially if you are older. You have been warned!

The key benefit of stretching muscles before you start walking is that this warms them up. Warm muscles are more elastic, and their stretching is more effective. If you are just starting a stretching and flexibility programme, repeat each stretching exercise three times and hold the stretch for a count of ten seconds. As your flexibility increases, hold the stretch for a count of 20–30 seconds and do five repetitions. Remember to breathe normally. Like all exercises, stretching takes more effort and frequency to improve from zero to a desirable level than it does to maintain a level. You should perform the stretching exercises three to five days per week to *increase* flexibility, but you only need to do them two to three days per week to *maintain* flexibility. You will doubtless be glad to hear that more than five days per week is not necessary!

The three key stretches

The muscle groups that contribute most to the walking gait are (1) hamstrings, at the back of the thighs (2) calf muscles, and (3) quadriceps, at the front of the thighs. If you're basically in a good state of health and all these muscles more or less work properly, it is important to stretch them thoroughly before doing any vigorous walking. Here's how you do this:

Hamstring stretch – Stand with one foot on a chair, a park bench or even the bumper of your car, with the toes of your elevated foot pointing straight up. Make sure both legs are straight and the knees locked. There is a tendency to bend the knee of the weight-bearing leg, but keep it straight at all times. Place your hands on your hips and slowly bend forwards, trying to touch your nose to the knee of your raised leg. You will immediately feel the tension in the hamstring muscles in your raised leg. Don't bounce. After the count of ten, straighten up slowly and reverse legs.

Calf muscles and tendons stretch – Stand with your feet about 46cm (18in) apart and 1m (3¼ft) from a wall (or a tree, if you are outdoors). Lean forwards with your back straight and place both hands on the wall or tree. Slowly bring your hips forwards while keeping your legs straight and your heels flat on the ground. There is a natural tendency for the heels to rise. Keep them down and you will feel the pull on the upper calf muscles in both legs. Hold this position for a count of ten (for beginners), then ease back with your hips. Repeat three times. A variation of this exercise will stretch the lower part of the calf muscles as well as the Achilles tendon. With your feet, hands and body in the same position as previously, slowly bend your knees as if you were going to squat, but be sure to keep your heels flat on the ground. You will feel the pull on the lower calf muscles and Achilles tendons. Hold for the appropriate count, then slowly rise. Alternate the lower stretch with the upper stretch for the appropriate number of repetitions.

Quadriceps stretch – You might not be familiar with these muscles, but they are the big group on the front of the thighs that is commonly known as the "quads". They might not be as big as they were when you were younger, but they still need stretching before any serious walking. Stand next to a wall or tree for balance. Reach back and slowly pull your non-weight-bearing foot up towards your buttocks until you feel the tension or a minor, dull ache in the front thigh muscles. Don't pull the foot up sharply. Hold for the appropriate count, then switch legs. You should ultimately be able to touch your heels to your buttocks. However if you have arthritis, or any knee problems, do the best you can and take what you can get out of the stretch.

There is no question that if you do these three stretches regularly you will get more out of your exercise walk and will function better in your normal daily walking. And bear in mind: the older you become, the more important stretching and flexibility are ...

Walking the Right Way

You would be amazed how easy it is to walk badly. Or maybe you wouldn't! By now you probably think you have seen every kind of walk there is: the "pimp roll"; the arrogant swagger; the young "Chav" monkey walk; the little old lady scuttling across the street like a crab ... Well, whatever the kind of walk, it is important to perform it correctly. Here's how:

Posture is all

If you intend to walk for exercise and in order to keep supple, then posture is without doubt the most important aspect to bear in mind. Getting your body lined up properly before you take the first step and keeping it lined up throughout your entire walk will give you a more rewarding, less fatiguing workout. It will also help you improve your posture during your normal daily activities. Good posture is important because it helps your body to function at top speed. It promotes efficiency of movement and endurance and contributes an overall feeling of well-being.

Next time you are out on the street, take a close look at people walking by. Most strollers tend to walk with their heads tilted down, looking at the ground right in front of them. Their shoulders are slumped and their stomachs are sagging. You can get away with walking like this if you are walking slowly, but you will find that, as the pace of the walk picks up, the requirement for good posture increases.

This is without doubt a good thing, for good posture is also good prevention. If you have poor posture, your bones are not properly aligned and your muscles, joints and ligaments all take more strain than nature intended. Poor posture can cause you fatigue, muscular strain and, after a while, even pain. This most commonly manifests itself in lower back pain. So to avoid this, let's get you properly lined up before you start your walking programme.

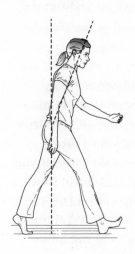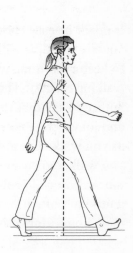

Look at the illustrations above. The first one demonstrates poor posture. Notice the vertical line of gravity and how the body is in front of that. The walker is increasing speed the wrong way: by literally falling forwards! The walker releases good toning tension on the lower abdominal muscles and transfers it to the lower back muscles, where it shouldn't be. The back muscles have to work harder to hold the torso forward of the vertical line of gravity. Unnecessary fatigue ultimately becomes discomfort and pain in the lower back. In the second illustration, notice the vertical line of gravity once more. This imaginary

49

line connects the ear, shoulder, hip, knee and ankle. It also passes through the hypothetical centre of mass. A properly aligned, healthy back has three natural curves: a slight forward curve in the neck, a slight backward curve in the upper back and a slight forward curve in the lower back. Good posture means keeping these three curves in balanced alignment.

It might be easy enough to maintain good posture when you are standing still, but it is another thing altogether to keep everything in the correct alignment when you are walking quickly. This takes practice and perseverance. Suffice to say that the fitter and more flexible your muscles and joints, the easier it will be to maintain good posture as you walk. The golden rule is to check your posture as you walk and ensure that you are not leaning forward too much. You will probably find that you often lean forwards a little too often; straighten up, and you will probably feel more comfortable right away.

Exercises *En Route*

Walking should be fun as well as keeping you flexible and fit, so you could try a few additional exercises to keep you amused as you wend your way along your walk.

As you become a more accomplished walker and start to pick up the pace, your upper body and the swing of your arms will become increasingly important. You will find that the faster you walk, the more you will need flexibility and looseness, particularly around the shoulder joints. As you begin your walk, loosen your arms and shoulders by swinging your arms across your body as if you were trying to wrap each one round your opposite side. Swing them with the right arm crossing over the left, then the left over the right. Swing them behind your back, so that the fingers of the opposite hands touch. You will feel your back and shoulders loosen up after a few swings.

As you continue to walk, swing your arms around like windmills a few times, clockwise and anticlockwise. Nice, easy swings will loosen up the shoulder joints for a freer arm swing during your walk. Roll your head around clockwise and anticlockwise several times to loosen up your neck muscles. All of this can be done simultaneously with walking and warming up your leg muscles.

If you really want to work on your flexibility while you are walking, you could also incorporate some of the general stretching exercises that are featured in the second chapter of this book. They will all make you feel good as you pick up your pace and become a better walker!

Walking Uphill and Downhill

A few nice, rolling hills will add variety to your walk and may or may not burn some extra calories into the bargain. It is probably not a good idea to start tramping up hills until you have become reasonably fit and a fairly accomplished walker, because this kind of walking understandably requires a greater effort than normal. It will certainly get the old heart working, but equally you want to be careful that it does not cause it to stop! If you walk up a hill, you have to walk down the other side, which burns fewer calories than walking up or walking on the level. If you wear a heart rate monitor, it is interesting to note how quickly your heart rate will increase when you are climbing a hill, even though your pace will slow, and then again how quickly it will start to drop as you crest the hill and head down the other side. Consequently, you will have to increase your speed considerably to keep your heart rate up when walking downhill. If one of your walking goals is to lose weight as well as to become more flexible and fit, you may find that when you average the up-and-down caloric expenditure of walking up hills, it may not be much more effective than that of a fast, sustainable pace on level ground.

The right technique
It might surprise you to know that there is actually a "right way" to walk up and down a hill. The Grand Old Duke of York and his 10,000 men might have got it down pat, but remarkably, maybe you have not!

Going uphill, one's first inclination (literally!) is to bend at the waist and lean into the hill. In fact that is wrong, and if you do so, you will soon have lower back muscles that are fatigued and hurting. What you should in fact do is maintain a proper erect posture and shorten your stride as you walk up the hill. Your pace will slow, but the pull of gravity as you go uphill will make you work harder, and your heart rate will actually increase. Remember that, when you walk up stairs, the average stair riser is only about 20cm (8in) high, so your step is automatically shortened. Keep your head up, your back straight from your ears to your ankles, and your shoulders over your hips. You can lean forward slightly by bending at the ankles, as race walkers do, but don't lose your posture. Walking downhill presents a different challenge. It is easy to maintain your posture, but how do you increase speed to keep your heart rate up without jarring your bones? Hold your body erect, almost as if you're leaning backwards, away from the slope of the hill. This is a good way to practise erect posture and it is easy to hold your head up. With your bent arms pumping fast to keep up with your accelerated leg swing, let gravity help pull you down the hill as fast as you can make your legs and feet move in a smooth, coordinated manner. This position also gives you a shorter leg swing, so that your foot doesn't have as far to drop down the hill at heel plant, and this reduces the jarring effect of downhill walking.

How Far Should You Walk?

So, if you have followed the advice in this chapter so far, you should be well on your way to becoming an accomplished walker. In the process you will undoubtedly improve your fitness, your flexibility and the strength of joints and muscles throughout your body. With any luck, you will also be feeling better about yourself, and everything else for that matter, as walking is incredibly effective at improving one's sense of well-being. Even for us wrinklies!

But what is the optimum distance to walk in order to gain the maximum benefit in all these areas of your health? Well, once again it all depends upon your level of fitness and mobility. Of course everybody is different and ageing affects all of us in different ways. Basically, it is up to you

– but, as with any form of exercise, it is important to build up the distance, duration and intensity of your walks in a steady fashion that is consistent with your level of health and fitness.

As a general rule, if you start off by walking for about 20 minutes and aim to cover at least 1.6km (1 mile) in that time, you could aim to build up to a daily walk of about 5km (3 miles) in one hour within several weeks. However, it is important not to overdo it. If you are in any doubt at all, consult your doctor before embarking on a programme of vigorous walking.

WALKING TIPS

- Wear sensible shoes. Brogues will do, but trainers or specially-designed walking boots are better – no matter how silly you might think they look!

- Avoid walking after a big meal. If you have just been enjoying *foie gras*, a steak in a rich sauce and a good bottle of Beaujolais, it might be tempting to try to walk it all off straight away. However, it is better to digest your meal properly before taking a post-prandial stroll – and avoid full-scale "yomping" late at night, as the general rush of blood and adrenalin will probably keep you awake in bed.

- Avoid walking during peak traffic hours – well, you wouldn't want to get run over, would you?! Ideally, find somewhere to walk that is far from the madding crowd and where you can breathe fresh air without fear or care.

- Take plenty of water. It is remarkable how much you can dehydrate just by walking, and this problem becomes worse as you get older. Sorry about that, but the fact is that lots of things do, don't they?

- Listen to your body. You might think "it's only walking", but it is still exercise, for which it is very easy to overestimate one's capacity … While the chances are that walking will only make you feel better, you don't want push it too far, so take your time and think W.G. Grace rather than Daley Thompson.

Conclusion

Who would ever have thought that a humble walk could do you so much good? Well, it will – but only if you do it properly, following the advice in this chapter to the letter. Remember, posture is all when walking, and maintaining a consistent pace while regularly increasing distance is the best way to increase both your levels of fitness and that elusive suppleness ...

Chapter 4

SWIMMING FOR SUPPLENESS

If you are looking for probably the best form of exercise in terms of improving suppleness, and you don't mind getting cold and wet, then try swimming. You might be put off by the idea of taking off your clothes in damp, draughty swimming pool changing rooms, yet once you've done this a few times you will get used to it and the chances are you will find that the benefits of swimming massively outweigh the disadvantages. Your body might no longer be the finely-honed, precision tool that it once was, and you might be self-conscious about the way it looks. But then again, maybe you don't care a jot! However, whatever state your body is in, what is certain is that regular swimming will improve both the way it looks and the way that you feel. You might look like Albert Steptoe rather than Johnny Weissmuller in your bathing suit. Your crawl might not be what it was as a baby. But you don't have to be a human otter to swim well and you're never too old to reap the benefits of this wonderful and uplifting activity. So, what exactly are they?

The Benefits of Swimming

There are so many reasons to take the plunge, old or young:

- Thirty minutes of steady-paced lane swimming burns over 200 calories – well over 400 in an hour.
- Any swimming that makes you breathe more heavily counts as "moderate" activity. Even treading water takes effort, so you are working most of the time you're in the pool. But remember – chatting with your friends in the shallow end only works your facial muscles!
- The pressure and resistance of the water makes your body work that little bit harder. Thirty minutes of activity in the water is worth 45 minutes of the same activity on land.
- The water takes your weight, so swimming can be great for those who want low-impact exercise – women during pregnancy for example, or for people who have mobility problems or want to protect their joints.
- Swimming works your whole body for all-over toning!
- Swimming is great for your heart. Because you are using your whole body your heart has to pump blood hard to your arms and legs, helping circulation too.
- Swimming is also great for your lungs – swimming lengths in particular forces you to breathe in a deep and

rhythmic way which gives your lungs a boost.

- Being in water can have great psychological benefits, too – the pool can "take you away from it all" and the feeling of being in water can be refreshing, relaxing and liberating as the water takes your weight.
- People of all different ages and abilities can enjoy swimming together – if you choose an activity you can do with friends and family, you are more likely to stick at it. You'll be having so much fun you won't notice you're working out, either!

So, it's a pretty beneficial form of exercise, whatever your age and condition. But the main thing about it is that – probably more than just about any other form of exercise – swimming will keep you supple!

What to Wear and Where to Go

One of the things that most puts people off swimming is the fact that it involves letting it all hang out in general view at the pool or the beach. For many individuals, whatever their age or degree of physical beauty, this can be an alarming prospect. However, for you, this may not matter. Perhaps age and experience have taught you that there are more important things in life than the state of your tummy or whether your legs look like Ginger Rogers' ... However, in all seriousness, as you become older there are other factors to consider about when and where to go swimming and what to wear.

THE RIGHT POOL FOR YOU

- Is there a suitable swimming pool nearby? You don't want to become exhausted by travelling miles before you even get there ...

- Does the local pool have scheduled times set aside for adults or older people? If you are embarking on a new swimming programme, you might want to avoid a crowd of screaming kids in the shallow end.

- Does your local pool offer suitable changing facilities for you? If you are in a wheelchair or need lots of room for any reason, it is worth thinking carefully about this.

- If you are in any way incapacitated or physically disadvantaged, does the pool you are intending to visit have easy access? You might actually need a mechanical hoist to get you into the pool. Most swimming pools have these nowadays, but it is worth checking in advance.

- Is the water warm enough? This might seem like a daft question, but some public swimming pools can feel like the River Volga in December, which might not suit your constitution. Another consideration is the amount of chlorine that is usually put into the pool in question. There is no point in going swimming if you're going to be seriously uncomfortable. You could always choose another form of exercise. Or just stay at home and have a cup of tea ...!

- Does your local pool offer swimming lessons? Maybe you need a refresher course or perhaps you simply haven't swum for years? Again, worth checking.

- Finally, is there a good snack bar you can retreat to for a warming cup of tea afterwards? You might just need it!

The gear you need

In the past a swimmer would emerge from the bathing hut
or carriage resplendent in a cover-all striped bodysuit –
perhaps with a straw boater on his head and an inflatable
duck under his arm to set off the look. Of course, we are
not seriously suggesting that you are that old, but times
have changed significantly, and now there is a whole range
of fancy new equipment that can make your swimming
experience more comfortable and enjoyable.

Starting from the top down, a bathing cap is definitely
a good idea if you value your coiffure. These days,
swimming pools tend to have so much chlorine in them
that it can destroy the hair of all but the youngest and
fittest. So, if you want to avoid your spouse commenting
on the strange, green, alien-like glow emanating from your
hair upon your return from the pool, invest in a cat.

Next, a decent pair of swimming goggles is an absolute
must. Select these carefully – don't just order them on the
Internet, but instead try on a number of pairs at the local
pool or sports shop – as you will feel as if someone has
tried to poke out your eyes with a blunt knitting needle
if you buy the wrong pair. Ill-fitting swimming goggles
can bring a whole new meaning to the term "sore eyes",
particularly for those whose sockets have been around
longer than most. Make sure that you tighten the elastic
on the goggles regularly, so that your poor old peepers
are not beset by an evil tide of chlorine every time you dip
your head in the water.

Now, here's the interesting part. Are you still sexy in Speedos? Would you look presentable in a pouch? Does your bikini still render you beautiful, or would you rather wear a gorilla suit than be seen dead in it? The choice, of course, is entirely yours – and what a huge choice there is to be had these days. Every conceivable kind of swimsuit – be it Bermuda, thong, mankini or fashion statement that beggars belief – is at your disposal, and just a click away on a website. But maybe, as with so many things, caution should be your watchword. A sensible, slick Lycra suit in a modest colour that keeps all your wobbly bits in place will probably be your best friend in the pool for an everyday swim for exercise and flexibility. Save the fancy stuff for your winter break in Barbados – or Bognor Regis ...

Warming Up for Swimming

Yes, it's that time again – the bit where we tell you all about the work that you have to do before you even start swimming! It's enough to make you head for the kitchen for another cup of tea ... But, as with all the forms of exercise featured in this book, you need to do at least some stretches and basic acclimatization exercises prior to beginning your swim. If you do not, you may continue to look more like Albert Steptoe and not at all like Johnny Weissmuller (he was an Olympic gold medal-winning swimmer back in the day, and then played Tarzan in the movies – remember?). And unfortunately there is no Cheeta to help you, either. So, let's start with some basic stretches.

The best way to warm up for swimming is to perform static stretches before you get wet. Static stretching minimizes the risk of injury and helps you feel stronger and "looser" in the water – whatever age you are and whatever your physical condition. If you're wondering how to swim effectively every day – or even just once a week – practise these pre-training static exercises. It might be a good idea to try them first in the comfort of your own home, so that you will feel less of a clot when you actually get to the pool. Ask your spouse what they think. Are you looking like Mark Spitz or Rebecca Adlington yet?!

Static stretches

Arm swings – The simplest and most common warm-up exercise for swimmers is the most important one you can do. Ten forward swings, ten backward swings and ten opposite direction swings will do it. If your arms feel like they're going to fall off, then make it five, and if you can't feel anything at all, then try 20 of each.

Hand slaps – Hold both arms straight out in front and swing one arm out to the side and then bring it back in front of you and slap your other hand to start it swinging out to the side. Have you ever seen the magnificent world champion swimmer Michael Phelps stand on the blocks and swing his arms behind his back? This warm-up exercise will really help you swim in the water. Ten hand slaps will do it.

Lunges – Walking lunges help warm up the legs for swimming, and help particularly with freestyle and freestyle turns. Keep your hips forwards and put pressure on the heels and not your toes.

Jump starts – Squat down with your hands in between your legs, and in your head say "Take your marks. Go" and on "Go" jump up to the sky in a streamline position. Practise five of these, working on jumping as high as you can. Make sure you don't land on the cat on the way down …

All these stretches – and any more that you feel might be beneficial – can be performed in your living room, in the changing rooms or at the poolside. The important thing is to do them immediately prior to beginning your swim. When you have finished, you can jump, lower yourself or climb primly down the ladder into the water. Now, don't take off as if there is an alligator after you, but instead take the time to perform a few water-bound exercises before you start swimming. This might seem like an awful lot of preparation to do before actually swimming, but your body will thank you for it later on.

Exercises in the water

Weightless walking – Walking in water is an ideal way to work on balance and to acclimatize to the water. Because it requires more energy expenditure, you can use the practice to burn calories. This exercise is particularly beneficial if you have joint pain and find it difficult walking on dry land. It is a great way to strengthen the leg muscles and exercise your joints without resistance while getting ready to swim.

Retro walking – Walking backwards in water, or retro walking as it is known, is a valuable form of exercise, which is becoming increasingly popular with physiotherapists as a part of rehabilitation programmes. This type of walking calls for an increased range of motion in the joints and a similar reduction of movement in the hip. Retro walking also requires more control of the trunk muscles, stretches the hamstrings and releases the hip flexors. You might feel like some antediluvian, aquatic version of Michael Jackson doing his famous "moonwalk", but this is a great way to improve your balance in the water, tone up your legs and pelvis and once again prepare for swimming.

Sideways stretching – Most people do not move sideways very often – leave it to the crabs – but in swimming it is an essential part of a couple of key strokes. Due to the reduction in frontal resistance, sideways movement through water is both easier as you experience the benefits of streamlining, and harder as it is more difficult to balance. Sideways movement is particularly important in front and back crawl, in which the aim is to minimize drag and maximize reach. Stand at full height and turn the body sideways with your feet together. Now elevate your left leg and step sideways, opening your arms to a horizontal level just above the surface of the water.

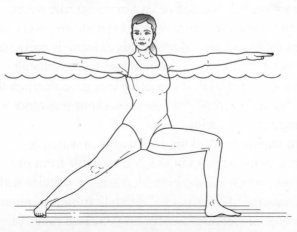

Okay, so you look like one of Busby Berkeley's Babes, but who's complaining! This movement should certainly make you feel more confident and buoyant in the water. Above all, it will get you used to the unnatural action of moving sideways.

The lunge – This exercise, which is performed in the water at the poolside, is good for spinal and general body alignment. It gives you the opportunity to free your neck and feel how your arm extension originates from your back. It also allows you to work on balance and stability in the water while your feet are still on the ground. Finally, it is a good way of making a smooth transition from standing upright to lying face down in the water. Stand in the water about 1m (3¼ft) from the edge of the pool. Place your right foot forward and gently release the knee. Try to keep both your heels flat on the floor. Keep your neck, back and head in a straight line as you press against the wall with the palms of your hands and send your back backwards. Remain in this position for a count of ten. Reverse legs and repeat the exercise.

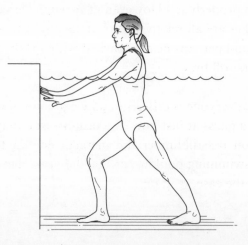

There are a great many other exercises you can perform prior to swimming, but if you just do the basics outlined above you will feel primed and ready to go. These exercises will make you feel great whether you swim or not! Depending on your level of fitness, and when you are starting out, you might decide that these are enough for one day and climb straight out of the pool ... Seriously though, now you're all set to swim!

Different Strokes for Older Folks

Perhaps when you were younger you would dive headlong into a cold pool and then simply hurtle up and down it for lengths on end, using a whole range of different strokes? Front-crawl, back-crawl, breast-stroke, English backstroke – all these and a few variations are within most confident swimmers' capabilities when they are young and fit. (You will notice that we have excluded the tricky butterfly stroke, which seemingly requires the aquatic skills and coordination of a duck-billed platypus in order to be performed properly ...) However, in varying degrees, these swim strokes are all relatively strenuous physical activities, which should perhaps be approached with a little caution as the years roll by.

Of course, everyone is different and we are not about to hazard a guess at just how fit – or not – you may be. Perhaps you are still limber and energetic enough to carry on in the swimming pool just as you did years ago but, if this is not the case, read on ...

Pace yourself

Successful swimming for suppleness and general fitness is all about working within your personal comfort zone – that is, not overdoing it – while changing the pace and mixing up your basic strokes and other moves to ensure that you receive the maximum benefit from the exercise.

Swimming will provide a complete body workout. Regular swimming improves endurance, muscular strength, posture, flexibility and the fitness of your heart and lungs. As we have seen, it is also a great activity for weight loss, as swimming at a medium intensity will have you training in your fat-burning zone, using up 200 calories in 30 minutes. When using the correct technique, swimming uses all key muscle groups, giving you an all-over body workout.

Front-crawl and backstroke give particular emphasis to toning shoulders, arms and stomach, while breast-stroke gives your thighs, stomach and buttocks a good workout. Alternate these with other moves, and you will maximize your health benefits.

Drills

You can do "drills" as part of your set (your swimming routine – see more on this below). This involves doing a length that is not using a recognized stroke but will help develop your technique and improve your stamina. For example, you can use a float to exercise arms only or legs only. You can swim breast-stroke with one arm only, keeping the other stretched out at all times. Or, swim front-crawl, but with only one arm cycling at a time, with the other stretched straight out in front.

Vary your pace

Try and avoid "plodding" as you move up and down the pool. Perform some lengths slowly, especially when you are "warming up". Then do some a little harder and then some as fast as you possibly can. This variation of pace will burn up calories and improve your stamina. Towards the end of your swim, swim a few lengths slowly as you "cool down".

Improve your efficiency

Occasionally count the number of arm strokes that you do per length and then try to reduce these. This will make your strokes more efficient. It will also keep you focused and the time will pass more quickly. You will soon find that you will be able to swim for longer distances within the time you have available.

Improve your stamina

Competitive swimmers train in "sets" and so can you. A "set" is performing a certain number of lengths and then stopping for a 20 second beak before continuing. For example, push yourself hard for two lengths and then take a break. You will build up your stamina by increasing the number of lengths you do in each set, as well as improving your suppleness.

Plan for variety

During your swim, plan to use a variety of different strokes. In addition to making the swim more interesting, it will give emphasis to different muscles, providing an all-over body toning session.

Set yourself goals

Whatever form of exercise you decide is right for you, it is always much easier to get fit and flexible if you set yourself goals. For example, you can set a goal for the distance you can comfortably swim in a set time in any particular stroke. When your original goals have been achieved, set new ones. You can reduce the time slightly or you can try and fit more lengths in the time you have. Be realistic, though – at first your goal may be just to make it to the pool twice a week!

Swimming With a Disability

If you have a disability, swimming might be the very best of all exercises to consider. Swimming is widely recognized as one of the best forms of therapy for people with disabilities. From the sensation of floating in water for the most severely disabled to actually learning to swim for the more able, water offers physical support that is greater than that provided by any other exercise medium, building confidence in those who enjoy its pleasures, no matter how physically disadvantaged they might be. Additionally, the movement of the body in the water gives a person with disabilities a sense of freedom, and for those with limited movement it can be used as an effective physiotherapy aid. Combine the health benefits and fun factor, and you can appreciate why swimming helps raise confidence and self-esteem for anybody with a disability, whatever their age and condition.

Many pools offer physical assistance to those with disabilities, as well as dedicated classes and pool sessions.

Check out what your local swimming pool has to offer and begin enjoying the amazing benefits of this most therapeutic form of exercise.

Aqua Aerobics

Swimming offers huge health benefits in abundance, as we have clearly seen, and in keeping with the main objective of this book, with regular practice it will keep you as supple as can be. However, for some people, after a while it can become ... well, a little ... BORING! All that ploughing up and down in lanes, while trying to avoid banging your head on the end of the pool and being splashed in the face by other swimmers – and you can't even wear an iPod while you are doing it! Now, we are not about to do down this most wonderful of activities, but we've said it: swimming can get a little dull after a while. But fear not – you don't have to abandon the pool just yet, for there is a wonderful alternative that any reasonably fit person of a certain age can try – aqua aerobics!

This alliterative aquatic activity (it's catching!) is not only a great way to get fit but is also one of the safest. It keeps the heart and lungs healthy while toning the body and reducing fat, and also provides a good opportunity for a general splash about in the water.

What is aqua aerobics?

As the name suggests, aqua aerobics is essentially aerobic exercise in the water. It typically takes place in shallow water at a swimming pool and as part of an organized group session that can last anywhere between 30 minutes and an hour. Workouts usually comprise of routines familiar to those who have experienced aerobics on land, and could include jumping jacks, cross-country skiing motion and walking and running backwards and forwards. Workouts also commonly feature such special water devices, such as "noodles" (nothing to do with Chinese food) or "woggles" (did you wear one of these at Cub Scouts?), which are used to aid flotation and resistance.

Safe exercise

The support the water provides for the body greatly reduces the risk of bone, muscle and joint injury, its density meaning that 90 per cent of a body's weight is supported. Another way to understand this is that a body weighing 68kg (10st 10lb), for instance, will only, in theory, weigh around just over 1st or 7kg (15lb) in the water. The stress that gravity puts on the body joints is therefore greatly relieved, enabling freer and safer movement. This water support also means that those with back or knee problems can take part in aqua aerobics without fear of pain or further injury. All this makes aqua aerobics an ideal, fun exercise for everyone with a basic level of fitness.

Water-based heart rate is approximately 13 per cent lower than during land-based exercise, due to the reduction of pressure, gravity and temperature on the heart that the water provides. Those with concerns about their hearts can therefore feel safer in the water, knowing that water-based exercise is relieved of much of the stress of most land-based exercise.

Not only does aqua aerobics welcome participants of a wide variety of sizes, and levels of fitness and health, but it is also open to non-swimmers, as the exercise is performed in chest-deep water. It is therefore one of the safest of all watersports.

Health benefits of aqua aerobics

As well as easing concerns over safe exercising, there are numerous health benefits to performing aerobic exercise in the water. Most significantly it increases cardiovascular fitness, promoting the service the heart provides in pumping blood around the body, and improving aerobic endurance. It also strengthens and tones the body and improves flexibility.

The density of water means that it provides 12 times the resistance of air, and therefore makes an exercise on land 12 times harder in the water. This means participants expend a good deal more energy than their cousins in the gym performing the same routines. The resistance also means that opposing muscle groups are strengthened by pushing against the water.

Nevertheless, much less is accomplished in a 30 minute period and so sadly aqua aerobics is not a major calorie burner. For instance, over such a period, aerobic water exercise could burn off around 300 calories.

Exercising in the water is also a great way to relieve stress, as the water massages and cools the body, relaxing you as you exercise.

Conclusion

Okay, it's wet, it can be cold and you have to show off
your body in public – well, at least a little bit – but then
again, swimming is incredibly good for you, great fun
and the king of exercises when it comes to suppleness.
The physical support that water offers means that just
about anyone can take part in this most liberating pursuit,
so unless you are allergic to chlorine or have got rabies,
swimming comes highly recommended.

Chapter 5

CYCLING FOR SUPPLENESS

Norman Tebbit said it years ago, of course – "On yer bike!" Now, he was talking about the fact that during the 1930s his unemployed father didn't give up, he got on his bike and looked for work and didn't stop until he found it, but switch the word "work" for "fitness" (or suppleness, if you want to be really pedantic), and the exhortation is just as valid in your case, 80 years on!

For cycling is one of the really fun forms of exercise that it is never too late to enjoy. You don't have to dress like a giant insect in a black helmet, with weird sunglasses, and lurid Lycra clothes; you don't have to try and be Lance Armstrong and win more *Tours de France* than you can shake a stick at; you just need a basic bike, a safe route and a bit of gumption, and you will soon be having a terrific time while getting fitter and happier into the bargain. So, take Norman's advice – get on yer bike!

The Benefits of Cycling

Cycling is a low-impact, aerobic workout that provides myriad health benefits. It is one of few forms of exercise that can be continued throughout life without involving a major time commitment or huge expense.

Numerous studies have found that cycling provides a variety of health benefits. Some of the benefits address specific health concerns, and others result in more general or indirect health benefits. These include:

- **Improved cardiovascular fitness** – Cycling strengthens the heart, which improves blood circulation and reduces blood fat levels and resting pulse. Riding for as little as 30 minutes every other day meets the British Heart Foundation's recommendations for a healthy heart.
- **Increased joint movement and less pounding** – Cycling reduces the risk of arthritis (or inflammation of the joints) caused by worn-out cartilage. This is one reason why it is a particularly good form of exercise for older people. Exercises like running put more stress on joints and break down cartilage, especially in the knees. On the contrary, cycling is gentler on joints and can actually strengthen them, because the cycling motion provides nourishment that builds up cartilage.
- **More active lifestyle** – Cycling (and other exercise) combats the dangers of a sedentary lifestyle, which increases the risks of cancer, heart disease, diabetes, osteoporosis and respiratory ailments. All of these diseases can be prevented – even reversed – with regular exercise. Further, regular exercise increases the heart's

ability to pump blood, even when you are sitting still.

- **Reduced back pain** – Cycling (and other exercise) provides nourishment that discs in the spine need for development. The large muscles in the back develop and become stronger. And cycling strengthens the small muscles that support individual vertebrae.

- **Stress reduction** – Moderate exercise, including cycling, reduces stress, which leads to lower cholesterol and blood pressure.

- **A stronger immune system** – Moderate exercise causes a boost in the immune system by increasing the production of cells that attack bacteria. Going for an easy bicycle ride can even make you feel better when you have mild cold symptoms without fever. This applies at any stage in your life.

- **Sweating** – Cycling causes most people to sweat, which is good for you because you sweat out toxins and (ideally) replace lost liquids with clean water.

- **Weight loss and fitness** – Any exercise, including cycling, burns calories, raises the metabolic rate and builds muscle tone, so you burn more calories while at rest. This can combat the well-documented effects of obesity, including increased risk of disease and early death.

- **Clean air** – Cycling is non-polluting and can help us breathe easier. Much of the pollutants and irritants in the air are the result of fossil-fuel emissions and can cause serious health problems, including asthma, irritation of the lungs, bronchitis, pneumonia, decreased resistance to respiratory infections, and even early death. These health risks are accentuated in children. When people ride bikes instead of driving cars, everyone's health benefits.

- **Ease of incorporating it into your life** – Cycling generally does not involve a steep learning curve and a lot of expensive equipment (beyond a bike and a helmet, other cycling gear is completely optional). In most areas, you can cycle year-round, and build it into your daily routine by cycling to work or doing errands. Most people can continue cycling indefinitely. This means that you will be more likely to stick with cycling than other forms of exercise long term, and lead a healthier life.
- **Exposure to sunlight** – Vitamin D generated from 15 minutes of sunshine a day can help prevent prostate cancer, breast cancer and osteoporosis. Having said that, of course too much exposure to sunshine increases the risk of skin cancer, so don't forget the sunscreen!

Buying a Bike and Getting Gear

Arguably the most enjoyable part of cycling is choosing and buying your bike – because these days, as with so many things, there is just so much choice! Of course, that might actually put you off – but if you are "into" machines generally, then you won't be disappointed when you go looking for a bicycle.

For a mode of transport that started out life as the pedal-less "boneshaker", followed by the unmistakable "penny farthing", the bicycle has come a very long way indeed. Now your metal steed of choice might feature as many as 30 different gears and might not be made of metal at all, but rather of some futuristic, impossibly lightweight fabric like carbon fibre or titanium. Strewn with "as standard" gadgets that you might associate more with

a spaceship from science fiction than the humble push
bike, your average bicycle is these days something of a
technological thing of wonder. And that's before you even
get started on the accessories you can buy for it!

For these reasons, this is not really the place to be
giving you detailed advice about which machine to buy.
Far better to head to your local chain of bike shop.
Alternatively, a trip to your local bicycle dealer will
probably yield fewer competitive deals but conceivably
a better and more individual choice of machine. Then
again, as with everything, the Internet can take you
places in bicycle world that you almost certainly did not
know existed – if you are so inclined and you know your
way around a PC keyboard and broadband connection.

Consider buying secondhand

If you have not ridden a bike for a number of years and
are not 100 per cent certain that this is the exercise of
choice for you, it might make sense to consider buying
a secondhand one – at least for starters. You could save
a fortune and you would be amazed at the number of
secondhand bikes out there. Lots of bicycle dealers offer
well refurbished and maintained used bikes. eBay is
positively swarming with the things because, just as Boris
Johnson seems to have realized in London with his rent-a-
bike scheme, these days everyone seems to want to emulate
"Daisy" from the old song and climb onto a bicycle,
whether it's made for one or two ...

If you do opt to buy a bicycle secondhand, *caveat
emptor*! If you don't know what that means (it's actually

"buyer beware!"), then maybe you are not as wrinkly as we thought and perhaps they had stopped teaching Latin by the time you got to secondary school ... Seriously, though, check any machine over thoroughly for wear and tear and basic operational functionality before parting with your cash, and then consider taking it for a thorough service before actually riding it.

Other gear

When it comes to other gear for cycling, all you really need is a helmet. Just don't fall for all the other mind-bogglingly expensive clothing, accessories and needless baubles that every cycle shop or department now seems to offer. If your goal really is suppleness and a little extra fitness – plus maybe the sheer pleasure of a ride in open countryside, if you want to make the most of this sport – then protect your head against a fall with a well-fitted helmet and forget about everything else. The non-stop fashion parade that the majority of the cycling world now seems to insist upon will merely encumber you and make you feel hot, sweaty and probably very self-conscious, when what you should be concentrating on is changing gear and avoiding potholes ... A good helmet can easily be found at any cycle shop and need not be expensive. Make sure it fits well and does not fall forward over your eyes when the straps are tightened – then it's chocks away for the main event!

Warming Up for Cycling

If you do it properly and with any real vigour, cycling will genuinely stretch and exercise muscles that you probably never even knew you had! For this reason, and also because your body is probably not as young and fit as it once was, it is essential to warm up properly prior to cycling. Some cyclists past the age of 50 or so have bodies of steel and might not see the need for a warm-up programme. However, with respect, the chances are that your body has seen better days and it will pay to stretch it thoroughly before you get on your bike.

THE BENEFITS OF A GOOD WARM-UP

A proper warm-up for cycling offers many benefits that prevent major injuries. These include:
- Thinning body fluids to allow easier muscle contraction and less work for the heart.
- Opening capillaries to bring more oxygen to the working muscles.
- Sensitizing the nervous system for smoother movements.
- Decreasing stress on the heart and muscles.
- Raising muscle temperature so contractions are more rapid.
- Conserving carbohydrates and releasing fat for fuel.
- Reducing initial levels of lactic acid.
- Helping asthmatics avoid constriction of airways.

The amount of warm-up required varies from one individual to another, but generally increases with age. A young cyclist may need only ten minutes of warm-up, whereas sadly a cyclist past 50 may require twice as much to realize the same benefits! It also depends what kind of ride you are preparing for. A gentle potter around the park obviously does not require as much preparation as that for a major trek over the hills and far away ...

Stretching

Something of a holy grail when it comes to exercise – particularly as you get older – stretching is vital for injury prevention. In fact, a lack of it is the main cause of physical breakdown in older people who exercise regularly. So, we now repeat the mantra that forms the backbone of this entire book: stretch, stretch, stretch!

You might feel old and stiff and the prospect of climbing onto a bicycle might actually fill you with horror, but it is important to realize that, whatever state you have got yourself into as you have become older, you can reverse the loss of flexibility that begins in most people as early as the fifth decade of their life. And the key to this is stretching.

Stretching methods have changed over the decades. In the 1960s, ballistic stretching with rapid bobbing movements was popular. Everybody bounced up and down like jackrabbits while believing themselves to be becoming fitter and more flexible. Well, nothing could have been further from the truth, because what is actually required for greater flexibility is static stretching. As we have seen elsewhere in this book, this involves holding a stretch for between ten and 30 seconds in order to realize the maximum benefit to the muscle being stretched. Before you climb on your bicycle, you should thoroughly stretch your hamstrings and quadriceps. Read the detailed descriptions on how to do this in Chapter 3, "Walking for Suppleness", on pages 46–47.

Weight training

If you are serious about your cycling and intend doing more than a few miles at a time on several outings per week, you should definitely consider doing some weight training in preparation. Once again, when it comes to basic strength and muscle mass, the spectre of age looms. Sadly, it happens to us all – we all lose both of them. Once you get past about 40, your muscles diminish in size and your bones simultaneously become less dense. This increases the likelihood of injury and, when it comes specifically to cycling, results in less power for sprinting or riding the bicycle up hills. Reduced bone health is a particular concern. Having said all that, the good news is that once again, the more active you are, the smaller the losses. This applies both to muscle mass and bone density.

Cycling is a great sport for maintaining lower body muscles and bones, but it does little for the upper body. If it is your sport of choice, it is important to do other exercise in addition – to work the upper half of your body, and prevent the health problems that can occur in later life, particularly osteoporosis. Weight training as a part of your regular cycling warm-up is one good solution. A few years ago, a university study conducted with subjects aged 55 and older found that combining weight training with a vigorous cycling programme improved bone density in both the upper and lower body areas.

The benefits of weight training

Besides improving muscle mass and bone density above the waist, weight training strengthens the muscles, tendons and ligaments of the foot, ankle, knee and hip joints that are so important to cycling. It can also correct imbalances and improve the range of motion of joints. All this means a lower risk of injury in the short term and later in life.

There are many different forms of weight training and tailored programmes galore. If you are serious about adopting this form of exercise as part of your cycling warm-up, then it is probably best to join a gym and employ a personal trainer to show you how to get the most out of using weights. Alternatively, you can buy your own set of weights and work out at home. The training will do your strength and flexibility no end of good, whether you are preparing for cycling or not. However, it is very important to appreciate that weight training itself can cause injury, particularly to older muscles.

Wherever and however you choose to weight train, bear the following basic rules in mind:

- **Train the big muscles** – These are the ones found in the thighs, bottom, calves, back, abdomen and chest. Use free weights for the best effects.
- **Use multi-joint exercises** – A multi-joint exercise is one that involves two or more joints within the same movement. For example, a seated knee extension works the quadriceps muscle on the front of the thigh, but uses only the knee joint. However, the squat also works the quadriceps, while including the knee, hip and ankle in the action. Because you use so many joints, you work more muscles at the same time. As well as the quadriceps, the squat exercise also strengthens the hamstrings, calves, gluteus and lower back.

- **Mimic the positions of cycling** – When doing the squat exercise, place your feet the same width apart as the pedals on your bike with your feet pointed straight ahead. This will help you to develop the strength you need to transfer to useable strength when you ride your bicycle.
- **Keep the number of exercises to a minimum** – Focus on performing several basic sets in a few key exercises rather than doing multiple exercises. By using multi-joint movements, you can greatly reduce the number of exercises you need to do in the gym. That means less time lifting and more time riding your bike!

Cycling Refresher Courses and Proficiency Tests

Suggesting that you need training to ride a bike might sound a little like a process involving education, grandmothers and sucking eggs, but if it has been a long time since you last climbed aboard a metal steed, perhaps this wouldn't be such a bad idea.

You might remember the Cycling Proficiency Test from your youth – yes, it's been going a surprisingly long time! First "road-tested" as long ago as 1947, the National Cycling Proficiency Scheme was formally introduced by the government in 1958, with statutory responsibility for road safety being given to local authorities in 1974, including the provision of child cyclist training. This scheme was aimed primarily at children, but anyone could take the test, in the interests of general road safety and to give cyclists some quantifiable idea of their standard of... well, proficiency. This served as a minimum recommended standard for cycling on British roads and was long regarded by children as something of a rite of passage (at least before they all discovered computer games instead ...). The test has now been superseded by the new National Standards for Cycle Training, branded "Bikeability" in England and launched by various cycling organizations in conjunction with the Department for Transport, which has its own distinctly garish website at www.dft.gov.uk/bikeability. There are three levels to Bikeability:

- Level 1 (red badge) covers basic bike handling skills and is delivered in a traffic-free environment, such as a playground.
- Level 2 (amber badge) is taught on quiet roads but in real traffic conditions and covers simple manoeuvres and road sense.
- Level 3 (green badge) covers more complex situations and equips the cyclist to handle a wide range of traffic conditions and road layouts.

Bikeability is an all-ages programme. The lower levels replace the Cycling Proficiency scheme, which as we saw above was targeted mainly at children. Levels 2 and 3 correspond to the skills delivered by the US Effective Cycling programme developed by John Forester.

Training for children and adults alike progresses through the three levels. This programme is now being delivered across the UK, usually with some form of government funding for training in schools and sometimes with subsidized or free training for adults.

So, if you haven't ridden a bike for a long time, consider brushing up your skills with this course. The website will tell you where you can find training locally. Don't be shy – plenty of older people take the course, and it might be a great way to meet some cycling companions.

If you don't feel like following a formal training course and think you might be a little long in the tooth for coloured badges you could instead contact one of the following cycling organizations to enquire about basic refresher courses:

- RoSPA
- LARSOA
- British Cycling
- CTC
- Sustrans
- Cycling England

These can all easily be found on the Internet, where dedicated websites will give you a thorough grounding in their particular services and cycling specialities.

The Best Way on the Bike

Going back to those grandmothers and eggs we mentioned earlier, in these pages we are not about to teach you how to ride a bicycle. That would be beyond the scope of this humble tome and, in any case, cycling is one of those things that you can't really learn from a manual – you just have to do a Norman Tebbit: get on your bike and figure it out for yourself!

Having said that, there is plenty of good advice to be had about the best way to approach cycling as a sport for increased fitness and flexibility in later life. Here is some of the best of it:

THE GOLDEN RULES OF CYCLING

- **Ride frequently** – The most basic element of health and fitness is regular exercise. Don't let your bike collect dust. Try to wear one out every four or five years. The more often you have to replace bikes, the healthier and fitter you will become.

- **Rest regularly** – Frequent riding demands a balance of regular resting. Keeping a balance between stress and rest is necessary for physical improvement – particularly as you become older.

- **Set challenging goals** – Expect nothing but the best from yourself, whether on or off the bike. Okay, that might sound like very American advice, but it is a good credo for any form of exercise, including cycling.

- **Believe in yourself** – Remember that you have a lot going for you as a veteran cyclist, especially the wisdom that comes from experience. Just because you are old doesn't mean you can't be a good cyclist!

- **Don't overreach yourself** – All right, we said set challenging goals, but equally you must be realistic about what you can achieve. If you overdo it on your bike, you will injure yourself, plain and simple.

Words of Wisdom and Warning

To boil it down to the three best and simplest pieces of cycling advice:

Rule 1 – RIDE CONSISTENTLY
Rule 2 – RIDE MODERATELY
Rule 3 – REST FREQUENTLY

To expand a little on these useful maxims, rule one is based on the premise that nothing does more to limit or reduce fitness than missed rides. If you're going to cycle and really want to feel the benefits in terms of greater flexibility and general fitness, then you must keep doing it regularly. Every interruption, whether caused by laziness, injury, burnout or illness will frustrate you – and you will stiffen up again in no time. So, if you choose this exercise, keep it up!

Riding moderately means exactly that. Keep to gentle terrain and manageable distances – not great hikes up hills and mountains! Cycling ceases to be enjoyable if it becomes too painful ...

Resting frequently will probably come fairly easily to you at your stage of life. Seriously, though, don't underestimate what a demanding form of exercise cycling can be. Take complete and proper rests to balance the physical demands of this wonderful sport and you will enjoy it all the more.

Warming Down After Cycling

Finally in this chapter, a word about warming down – or cooling down, if you prefer the older, less technical and probably more accurate description of this important component of most exercise.

Cooling down after cycling is actually very important – if you want to avoid pulled muscles and aching joints. Cycling is a fairly intense form of exercise in which many muscles and joints receive a pretty strenuous workout, particularly in the legs, backside and pelvis. The other thing to bear in mind is that, as cycling is an outdoor activity, you might undergo an extreme change of temperature as you depart your saddle for your armchair (or bath), especially if you are riding in winter. This can be an unpleasant and potentially painful shock for old body parts as well!

The best way to cool down after cycling is to do exactly what you did to warm up! Turn back to the beginning of this chapter and revisit the various stretches that are discussed. Alternatively, try just about any of the other stretches covered elsewhere in this book – although we would not recommend a full session of yoga immediately after a ten-mile ride!

The key thing is to avoid massive drops or increases in temperature – by removing or adding articles of clothing as soon as you climb off your bike – and to ease out muscles that have been worked harder than usual and that contain a higher level of lactic acid than they are used to. Spend 10–15 minutes letting your body gently re-acclimatize to being back on *terra firma* as opposed to on two wheels, and you will notice the benefits in the morning. You will also find it a lot easier to climb back onto your bike the next time.

Conclusion

Cycling is one of those sports that, if you take it up, you will never let go. There is something wonderfully compulsive about this form of exercise that only ever makes you feel really good whenever you do it. It might not be the best workout for the upper half of the body, but it will give you all the cardiovascular fitness you will ever need while keeping your legs, backside and pelvis in tiptop condition. For all-round suppleness and fitness training, combine it with some weight training and the upper body stretches featured in Chapters 2 and 7.

Chapter 6

YOGA FOR SUPPLENESS

As you get older, you become stiffer and less supple – it's just one of the inevitable facts of ageing, like an expanding waistline and forgetting where you left the car keys. You know you should do something about it – go to the gym, join an aerobics class – but it's so much easier simply to collapse in front of the telly with a glass of wine and a sandwich. After all, you could always just watch sport … just like the man in your life.

However, if you really want to start easing up those creaking joints and aching muscles you could always try yoga. This centuries-old mind and body workout from the Far East is no longer the preserve of weird hippie types or pretentious yummy mummies from trendy suburbia. No, these days everybody's doing it – and it even works for us! There are hundreds of different poses, exercises and routines to choose from and you don't need much in the way of equipment. Fifteen or 20 minutes a day is all it takes to make a fairly noticeable difference to your fitness – in particular your flexibility and general suppleness – no matter how unfit you may have become. The following pages offer you advice on getting started, a range of tips especially tailor-made for yogis of greater vintage, and a number of classic yoga "asanas" or postures that won't break either your back or the bank. Make these exercises part of your weekly routine and, who knows, you might even feel the years fall off you. If not, you can always re-join your other half in front of Sky Sports.

Yoga for Flexibility, Balance and Strength

If you are looking for a low impact, quiet and peaceful form of exercise that you can perform either in the privacy of your own home or in the security of a supervised class, yoga could be for you. However, if you have arthritis, rheumatism or any significant mobility issues, then it's probably best to look elsewhere in this book, but if not, read on.

Flexibility

Getting fit and flexible again is not just about how fast you can run or how much weight you can lift. There are many components to fitness and flexibility – or suppleness, if you prefer – is just one of them. Your flexibility is your ability to bend – your range of movement around a joint. Flexibility can be both maintained and improved through stretching and yoga can help you to achieve just that.

If the body is not regularly taken through its full range of movement, then you will experience a loss of flexibility. This is particularly true as you become older, so it's especially important for people of our age to pay attention to the various siren calls of their bones, joints and muscles.

Additionally, imbalances in the body may be introduced through a lack of specific exercise or training that together can increase the risk of muscle injury and muscle pain, such as back pain, which is particularly common. Without regular training, the muscles will often shorten and permanent loss of flexibility can occur. The earlier in life one starts training, the more these negative effects can be delayed or indeed reversed, as everyday movements alone will probably not be sufficient to take your body through the range of movement it needs to remain fully supple. However, if you are coming to this awareness relatively late, do not despair – the human body's capacity for rehabilitation and renewal is really quite remarkable, even when it has begun its slow and creaky descent into old age.

Practise regularly

If you are planning on taking up yoga, be aware that it is important to perform the exercises very regularly in order to realize lasting physical benefits, especially improved flexibility. Any breaks in regular yoga training will quickly result in a loss of flexibility, but keep it up and improving your flexibility will help you to feel younger for longer.

Some are more supple than others ...

There is a huge amount of variation in peoples' flexibility, as you will be able to see whenever you attend a yoga class. Everybody has their own unique physical history and this has a distinct bearing on their specific level of flexibility. Simple things like how you sit each day, which activities and sports you do and any injuries that you have had in the past, can all influence your flexibility – so no two individuals will ever be exactly alike. Don't be discouraged if you find at first that you cannot do simple exercises that you would have been able to perform easily when you were younger, such as kneeling or turning your head to look behind you. Everybody feels the ravages of time in some way. Rather, take comfort in the fact that, with practise, your old abilities will probably soon return – and congratulate yourself for being a go-ahead yoga devotee and not some sit-at-home stick in the mud!

Strength

Strength is a component of fitness that is not immediately associated with yoga, which most people think of as a languid, tranquil sort of activity. However, when it comes to practising yoga, lack of strength can easily be the sole reason for not being able to master a pose. Unfortunately it is not enough to be able to get into a pose for a second or two – you must be able to hold and feel comfortable in the pose in order to have truly mastered it. Positions such as the plank pose (see page 130) require a great deal of body weight to be supported on the arms and hence fairly significant arm strength is required. In fact, strength is needed to enable you to hold many of the exercises featured in this chapter. Again, though, if you are reading this as you are just starting out, don't despair. Keep practising gently and slowly, without pushing yourself too hard, and the strength will come. Try some of the other stretches and forms of exercise discussed elsewhere in this book as well and it will come even quicker!

Balance

Balance, like strength, is also not generally associated with yoga. However, a lack of balance can also easily be the sole reason for not being able to master a pose. Good balance is required to enable you to hold several of the exercises presented in this chapter, so if you get dizzy just climbing out of the armchair, have a chat with your doctor before deciding to take up yoga. Having said that, if you are confident in your basic abilities and level of fitness, just keep practising your balance by holding these poses for increasing amounts of time. Better balance, like improved strength and flexibility, will come the more you practise yoga. And you will feel proud of yourself whenever you master one of the more demanding poses!

There are a few basic techniques you can use to start training your balance, such as:

- Focusing your gaze on a steady point.
- Slightly bending at the knees as you begin an exercise.
- Widening your base by placing your feet further apart.
- Supporting yourself against a wall.

Getting Started

You will need your own space in which to practise yoga – ideally a warm, airy room – no howling draughts or dogs. The basic equipment required to get started is a yoga mat, two yoga blocks and a yoga belt. These can be purchased inexpensively from most sports retailers or via the Internet from one of the many specialist yoga suppliers. A blanket will also be useful – if you collapse in a tearful heap halfway through your routine, you can always wrap it around you. Now all that is required is a little discipline and the setting aside of a regular time to practise. You might be getting on a bit, but chances are you still have a hectic life; however, do try to avoid telling yourself that you are too busy to find time to practise regularly. Yoga pays dividends pretty quickly, so it is worth persevering. By becoming fitter, healthier and more focused, your efficiency level will improve and you will very soon find you have more energy. As a result, your coping skills will receive a boost, enhancing your enjoyment of life and improving your general productivity, whether it is in your work, your leisure or your family life.

TOP TEN YOGA TIPS

1 Consult your doctor before you begin to practise yoga – Jane Fonda in *Barbarella* you might once have been, but you are not now!

2 Try to create the same space in your home to practise every day. Kick out the cat, the grandchildren and your spouse – this is your space!

3 Always use a proper yoga mat, as there is a real risk of slipping on any other surface – and you don't want any embarrassing breakages.

4 Wear loose, comfortable clothing and always practise yoga in bare feet – it'll make you feel like a proper yogi. The long, grey beard is optional, though.

5   Create a relaxing atmosphere. Light a candle or burn
    some incense. Now we're getting sensual …!
6   Turn off your telephone and television. Play some
    gentle music instead. Probably not Tom Jones.
7   To start with, set yourself a goal to practise yoga for
    15–20 minutes daily. Remember, you have to be able to
    walk around the rest of the week.
8   Don't forget to breathe while you practise yoga – in
    fact, that's probably a good general rule of thumb.
9   Try to stay in the present moment. Don't let your mind
    wander, as it might distract you.
10 Be aware of how you are feeling each time you start
    your practice. Don't worry if you can't feel anything at
    all – that means the exercises are working!

Your level of ability

Yoga is not a competitive sport, so you don't need to have
a certain level of flexibility in order to take part. The other
good piece of news is that yoga is suitable for all levels of
ability. In fact, the stiffer you are, the more potential benefit
you have to gain from yoga! If you decide to join a yoga
class, do not be disheartened by people around you who
may be more supple and able. View them as sources of
inspiration and allow them to show you the benefits that
they have enjoyed – especially if they are the same age as
you! (Seriously, many sports centres offer yoga classes that
are specifically reserved for older people.) Your current level
of ability will be determined by many factors, including:

• The range of motion you use in your day-to-day life.
• The physical activities you are currently involved in.

- The other activities you have been involved with in the past.
- Whether you have had operations or injuries.

Starting yoga will quickly show you the areas in which you are well developed and other areas that require more work. Don't shy away from what you learn about yourself. Instead, use this information to guide your training so that your body can become better balanced over time.

Your range of motion

The range of motion of your muscles is the range between the muscle being fully extended to that when it is fully contracted. In order to maintain your current range of motion, you need to take your body through this full range regularly – right across the whole body. This will help you to maintain both the extendability and the elasticity in your muscles. Without such regular training, the muscles will gradually shorten and this will alter the function of the joints and could also put undue stress on other parts of the body, leading to injuries.

Through stretching and yoga exercises you can work towards maintaining and even improving your range of motion, whatever your age and physical condition.

Your personal yoga development plan

The handful of exercises and poses offered below are presented as a basic introduction to yoga, nothing more. All the postures described are based on a step-by-step approach and are carefully designed to give an older, probably less flexible person, a good grounding in the principles of the art. Closely follow the step-by-step instructions and identify which step you can reach in any given exercise; then, use the progressive steps to track your progress. The key thing is not to push yourself too far, too fast and not to overreach yourself – remember you're just not as flexible as you used to be ...

Having said that, whatever you do, KEEP GOING! Taking even a couple of weeks away from yoga practice will leave you feeling stiffer than normal, which ironically is a good indication of the benefits you have been receiving through your training. Sadly, this problem becomes more and more acute as you get older. If you attend classes containing a mix of age groups, you will be able to see some of the effects that ageing has on the range of motion. Children tend to be very flexible, easily performing difficult exercises such as the lotus pose without effort. Similarly, older people may find that even some of the simplest exercises designed as part of the warm-up are difficult – for example, the neck and arm stretches. The only way to overcome this is to keep training regularly – without breaks!

Practising Yoga

To reap the full benefits of yoga, you must have patience and perseverance. If you think about it, these virtues sort of go with the territory. All that Far Eastern mystical focus and concentration, meditation and spiritual development ... "Patience and perseverance" might seem a little more prosaic, but you could view these qualities as modern Western equivalents of the original Eastern objectives in yoga! Seeing improvement in your yoga ability will be a slow, gradual and often surprising process. Do not expect just one or two sessions or lessons to show marked progress: it may take four or five good goes before you begin to feel any improvement. Remember – yoga training is not a race, even if as an older person, you feel you might be up against it time-wise. You must be patient and allow your body the time it needs to develop and grow stronger.

- Practise regularly so that your strength and suppleness increase steadily.
- Make movements slowly and safely – don't "snap" into positions!
- Don't go too far too quickly – if you over-reach yourself, you will get injured.

Do it often!

This is your yoga mantra: PRACTISE REGULARLY! Two to three times a week should certainly be enough to start to show you some benefits. As explained above, remember that any breaks in training will inevitably result in you feeling stiffer. However, as you become accustomed to it, yoga will become something that merges more and more into your everyday life, affecting how you sit and how you feel when you move.

When starting in yoga, you may well find that there are few poses you can achieve completely and comfortably. This is not a problem. It only indicates that you must first work on the preparatory positions that will eventually enable you to achieve the full pose. Too many yoga students try to go too far too quickly. This will only result in pain and perhaps even injury, and it will not aid your training as it may mean that you want to, or even need to, take time out. You must be patient with your body.

Moving in and out of positions should be done slowly and safely. If you are unsure about how fast to move, then a useful indicator is to time your movements with your breathing, which should be deep and relaxed. To get the most out of your practise, you should feel a stretch in the muscles that you are working. This may feel slightly uncomfortable, but it should be a good discomfort, which means that your muscles are working at the right level. You should not feel pain. If you do begin to feel pain, then you must either come out of the pose or make the pose slightly easier for yourself by pulling back a little or even moving back to an earlier step in the sequence. Pain and injury will not aid your training – they will only hinder it. Once a particular pose has been mastered properly, it will become effortless and cause no discomfort.

Yoga Training and Warm-up Tips

Here are some basic guidelines and rules of thumb that will make your yoga training more comfortable and beneficial:

- Do not practise yoga immediately after a heavy meal.
- Do not practise yoga on an empty stomach as your muscles work better when they are supplied with sufficient nutrients.
- Do not practise yoga after being out in the hot sun for several hours – you might get heat exhaustion.
- Be sure to have a short period of relaxation after each practice.

- If possible, have a shower both before and after yoga training to refresh yourself.

Here are some tips to help you during training:

- Your breathing should be comfortable and not restricted.
- Try to breathe through your nose rather than your mouth.
- Where a position is shown using one side of the body, make sure that you practise on both sides.
- It is better to hold a slightly easier position for longer than to push your body into a difficult position that you can hold for only a few seconds.
- If you are in a lesson, sit out any exercises that you are uncomfortable with for any reason.
- Pay attention to instructions during lessons, especially if they are anything to do with safety.
- Always keep a bottle of water near you during yoga training.

Words of Warning!

Attention! There a number of things you should bear carefully in mind whenever you are taking up yoga training, particularly as a citizen of the more senior variety. We hate to labour the point, but if you have any pre-existing medical condition, you should seek advice from a medical professional before beginning any training regime. Additionally, in particular, it is important to take note of the following:

- If you have high blood pressure, suffer from dizziness, have displacement of the retina or suffer from pus in the ears, avoid inverted poses and take extra care during any form of yoga exercise.

- Avoid compressive poses if they make you feel uncomfortable.
- Avoid inverted poses during menstruation.
- No undue stress should be felt in the head. Stop if you get pains in your cranium.

In general, the best way to practise yoga is to do only the poses that you are comfortable with. If a certain pose is too difficult, then it is better to find an easier version that you can manage rather than placing undue stress on your body. When training in a yoga class, do not feel under any pressure to try to "keep up" with other students. Just sit out any exercises that you are not confident about and do not wish to try. Yoga practice is not a competition. The most important thing is to train at your own pace and give your body the time that it needs to become comfortable with the poses.

Reclining Postures

Poses that require you to lie on your back can be greatly relaxing – but do try not to fall asleep! This section begins with the corpse pose, also known as the dead pose – but don't take either of these terms too literally … This exercise, although physically simple, requires much concentration and focus in order to steady your mind – which probably needs it. This exercise is commonly used at the end of the class in relaxation sequences. It can equally be used in between more demanding poses in order to allow the body and mind to be refreshed before progressing to more challenging poses.

The knees to chest pose is another exercise that can be used for relaxation. It has a great sense of rejuvenation about it, as the gentle twists in the body help to relieve any stress in the back. The last pose in this section is more difficult. The supine hand to toe pose focuses on working the legs, the hamstrings and the inside leg respectively, and you could feel as if you have been ten rounds with Mike Tyson after doing this one, so take it easy!

THE CORPSE POSE

This exercise is also commonly known as the dead pose or the resting pose. Although it looks simple, it is no excuse to have a sleep! This pose is an excellent one for working on being able to steady your mind. During this exercise, you should focus on sequentially and actively relaxing the muscles throughout your body. Practise slow and deep breathing and try to free your mind of all external concerns. Many yoga instructors use the pose to either start or end lessons. It helps to prepare the mind ready for the class and to relax you before you go back to your daily activities.

1 Lie on the ground with your arms resting naturally by your side and your legs comfortably apart. Try to rest

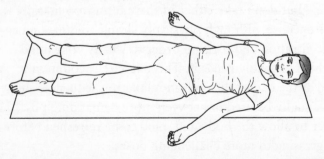

your sacrum (the base of the spine) on the ground. Let your feet lie in a natural position. Focus on successively relaxing each part of your body and letting it sink into the ground.

KNEES TO CHEST POSE

This exercise gently works the spine. It is another great exercise for using in a relaxation sequence or for punctuating between more demanding poses. Focus on letting the muscles in your body relax during this pose and let your breathing become slow and deep. Repeat this exercise several times, taking your time to move from one side to the other.

1 Lie on your back, keep your feet together and bring your knees towards your chest. Place your arms straight on the ground, in line with your shoulders. Your palms should be flat on the ground.
2 Rest your knees onto the ground on one side, keeping your shoulders flat on the ground. This move adds a gentle twist in the back.

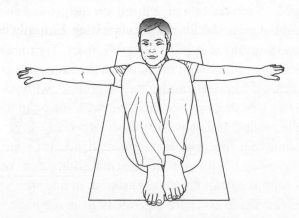

SUPINE HAND TO TOE POSE

This simple-looking exercise can be quite challenging. It works the abdomen and the muscles in the legs. Perform this exercise by slowly moving into the pose, holding and then out again. You may wish to use a strap for this exercise, if you are unable to reach your feet. Remember to practise this exercise equally on both sides.

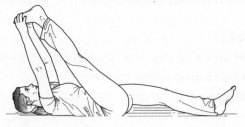

1 Start in the corpse pose.
2 Pull your feet back and ensure that your legs do not rotate away from the centre line. Bring one knee into your chest and hold it with your hands. Keep the other leg as straight as possible.
3 Bring your hands to your raised foot and then straighten your leg. Pull your leg in as close to your upper body as possible. Keep the other leg firmly on the ground and as straight as possible. Do not let your body lean over to one side or the other.
4 Holding your foot with the hand on the same side as your raised leg, rest your leg on the ground, with your other arm resting on the other side, with the palm flat on the ground, in line with your shoulder.
5 Holding your foot with the opposite hand, rest your leg on the ground, with your other arm resting on the other side, with the palm flat on the ground, in line with your shoulder. This move adds a gentle twist in the back.

Standing Poses

Standing poses are particularly good for strengthening the legs and practising your balance. Wrinkly beginners may find these exercises quite difficult, however, although many of them can be modified to make them achievable for newcomers until they have developed more by using the step-by-step approach presented here.

TREE POSE

This exercise will help you to work on your balance as well as your flexibility. Also it will require you to be able to lift your foot, unsupported, to the top of your thigh. It is best to work your way through the steps and stop when you reach the stage that you feel needs some work. It may be your balance or your ability to raise your leg unsupported that holds you back from achieving this pose. Step 3 is the simplest form of this exercise. It is best to focus here until you are able to balance, before moving on.

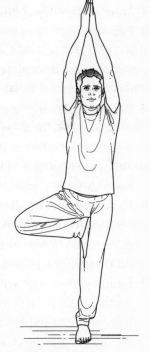

1 Start in the basic standing position. Keep your back straight and your shoulders down and pushed back slightly so that your chest is opened up.
2 Bring your palms together and then raise your arms above your head. Straighten the arms.

3 Lift one foot up and rest it on your ankle. Ensure that your toes point downwards and that your knee points out to the side.
4 Raise your foot and rest it on your knee. Again, ensure that your toes point downwards and that your knee points out to the side.
5 Raise your foot further and rest it on the inside of your upper thigh, reaching as high as you can. Keep your gaze parallel to the ground and focus on balancing in this position.

FORWARD BEND POSE

This pose works the muscles in the back of the body intensely. In addition, this standing version requires you to balance in position. Since it also results in inverting your head, if you feel any uneasiness when performing this exercise, you must stop immediately and speak to your instructor, if you have one. If you are unable to reach the ground in this exercise, then you should stop at step 3 and work towards lowering your upper body further before attempting the remaining steps. You can also try using blocks to give you support.

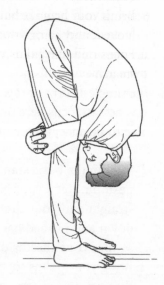

1 Start in the basic standing position.
2 Lift your arms straight above your head and stretch upwards, keeping your feet flat on the ground. You should feel your back and shoulders extending.
3 Interlock your fingers and, keeping the knees locked, bring your upper body downwards by bending at the waist. Keep the muscles in the upper body relaxed and let your weight bring you down.
4 Slowly reach further down and place your palms flat on the ground in front of you and about a hip-width apart. Bend forward from the pelvic region rather than the upper back and neck.
5 Reach through between your feet and rest your palms on the ground behind your feet. Try to bring your wrists in contact with your heels and point the fingers backwards.
6 Bring your arms behind your legs, keeping the knees locked, and bring your hands to rest on your elbows. Focus on your balance and keeping your breathing steady.

TRIANGLE POSE

This pose works the back of the leading leg and also develops your awareness of alignment and posture. If you are unable to reach the ground in step 3, then you could attempt this exercise with the use of a block under your hand. These various steps can be joined together into a sequence of increasing difficulty. The variant described subsequently is slightly more difficult than step 3, since it requires a slight turning of the upper body in order to place the hand on the other side of the foot.

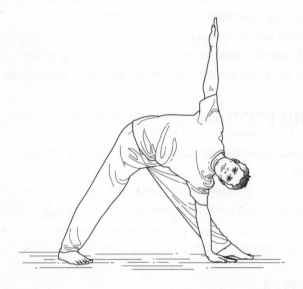

1 Start with your feet about two to three shoulder-widths apart (you want to form about 90 degrees with your legs), your back straight and your shoulders relaxed. Your toes should point forwards. Raise your arms to bring them in line with your shoulders and pointing out to the side. Your palms should face down.

2 Turn your feet to point to the side and look along your
  leading arm. Your leading foot should point directly
  forwards and your rear foot should point about 45
  degrees off to the side, so that it is in a natural position.
  Keep both legs straight.
3 Bend your upper body sideways and rest your palm
  flat on the ground with the fingers pointing forwards,
  alongside the inside of your leading foot. Your other
  arm should point vertically upwards and be in line with
  your supporting arm. (Repeat on the other side.)

Variant: Place your palm flat on the ground with the fingers
pointing forwards, alongside the outside of your leading foot.
Your other arm should point vertically upwards and be in
line with your supporting arm. (Repeat on the other side.)

Sitting Postures

The seated exercises presented below range in level of
difficulty, starting off with easier exercises and moving
on to more challenging poses. Despite being in a seated
position, these exercises will enable you to work the whole
body. They are particularly good for working on the
hamstrings, the hip adductors and the back.

STAFF POSE
The most basic sitting position is with your legs stretched
out straight in front of you. This simple exercise helps
to raise your awareness of how you sit and your overall
posture. Many yoga poses use this pose as a starting
position and then work on moving the rest of the body
into the correct position. Make sure that your back is

straight and that your knees are not bent. Do not let your hands rest on the floor behind you. Instead, place the hands lightly on your legs or in front of you. This will help to ensure that you keep your back straight and upright and remain balanced. Varying the position of the feet will vary the muscles that are engaged during this stretch. For example, if you pull your feet back then you will engage the hamstrings and the calves. If you point the feet, then you will feel the muscles on the front of the legs working. The further apart you push your feet, the more you will engage the hip adductors.

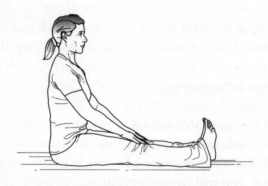

1 Sit with both legs straight out in front and your knees, heels and big toes touching. Push the back of your knees into the ground and do not let your legs rotate outwards. Place your palms flat on the ground either side of your hips and with your fingers pointing forwards. Keep your back straight and your shoulders down and pushed back slightly so that your chest is opened up. Push your pelvis slightly forward and bring your navel in slightly towards your spine. Hold your gaze parallel to the floor.

HEAD TO KNEE POSE

This literally-named pose brings the head down to rest on the knee. The exercises in this section are excellent for developing the back of the legs and the back. This is the starting position for a number of variants that can form a nice sequence. The bending must be done from your hips and not from the middle of your back or your neck. If you find that you are using your neck, make sure that you look towards your feet instead of looking at your knees and this will help to reduce the strain on your neck. It should also help to reduce the risk of bending forward using your back.

The exercise begins with the staff pose (see above) and works your hands gradually forwards, increasing the stretch in your back and your legs as you go. Each step represents an increasing level of difficulty. Work your way through the steps and stop when you feel you have reached a comfortable stretch. You can use these steps to give an indication of your flexibility for this particular exercise. Each step will also help you to map your progress over time. You will want eventually to be able to reach step 4 and rest your head down and feel comfortable in this position, reaching your heels with absolute ease and breathing without any feeling of constriction. The two variants shown are of increasing difficulty.

Step 3, where you cross your hands over and hold your shins in order to help control the amount of stretch, is a good place to stop if you cannot reach your heels. Slowly increasing how much you bend at the elbow in this step will increase the stretch.

1 Start in the staff pose.
2 Tuck one leg in so that your knee points out at 90 degrees. Ensure that your back is still straight by tilting your pelvis forward and pulling back your shoulders slightly to open up your chest.
3 Reach forward towards your foot, cross your arms over and rest your hands on your shins. Then bend your elbows in order to increase and control the stretch. Try to bend forward from the pelvic region rather than from your upper back or neck. This will become easier with practice. Keep your gaze parallel to the ground.
4 Reach further forward and hold the heel of the outstretched leg in your hands and rest your head down. Extend through the centre of your back and also your shoulders. Do not use your neck to pull you down.

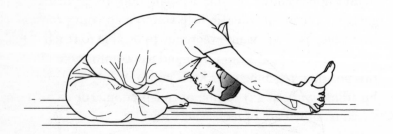

REVOLVED HEAD TO KNEE POSE

This pose changes the focus of the head to knee pose from just being on the posterior of the body to also working the side of the upper body. The final step leaves you in a comfortable and closed pose. Each step represents an increasing level of difficulty and so you should work your way through and stop at the appropriate level.

1 Start in staff pose.
2 Tuck one leg in so that your knee points out at 90 degrees. Ensure that your back is still straight by tilting your pelvis forward and pulling back your shoulders slightly to open up your chest.
3 Turn your body from your lower abdomen to bring the side of your upper body in line with your outstretched leg. Hold you arms up above your head and lean one arm towards the opposite leg. Try to bend along the side from the pelvic region rather than from your upper back or neck. You should feel a stretch in the side of your upper body.

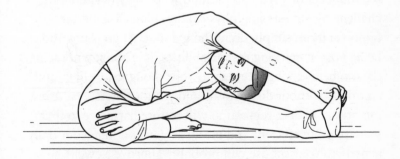

Rest Postures

When you have completed the active part of your yoga practice it is a good idea to rest for a short time so that you can enjoy and appreciate the sensations of well-being that (should!) have developed as a result of your training. It is a time to cool down and settle your mind before continuing with whatever is happening next ...

The secret of good relaxation is in the ability to "let go". Contrarily, these days, we all seem to be "on the go", all the time. Constant, relentless activity has become the norm in the West, whereas yoga was developed thousands of years ago by Far Eastern monks and spiritual gurus who had a very different take on the world and how to live in it (probably a much better one, frankly – all things considered!). The idea of "non doing" can be a difficult concept in our Western culture, in which being busy and continually active equate with importance and high status. Yet this approach denies the joy of freedom that the founders of yoga had in mind when they devised their challenging yet relaxing physical discipline. Taking the opportunity to simply do nothing and to let go is not about being lazy or shirking responsibilities. It is about embracing the moment, giving free rein to your thoughts, feelings and emotions without distractions and without pressures. A few minutes of proper relaxation will restore harmony so that you are more efficient and useful as you continue your daily activities. Your spouse will probably approve as well!

To wind down after your yoga session, lie on your back in corpse pose (see above) for two to three minutes or longer.

Exercise tends to raise the body temperature and this may fall quite quickly as you relax. You may wish to put on your socks or a jumper or, if you are lying down, perhaps cover yourself with a blanket.

1 Bring awareness to the contact that the back of your body is making with the mat to include the back of your head, shoulder blades, trunk, pelvis, legs, calves and heels. Feel the support underneath your shoulders, arms and hands. Surrender to the gravitational pull on your body as if you are sinking into the ground. Let go. Allow yourself to experience the sensations of being supported, grounded, down to earth. Stay with and embrace these sensations for several breaths.

2 Shift attention to your body surface. Allow the muscles of your face to soften, relaxing your eyes, eyelids, bridge of nose, cheeks, lips and root of your tongue. If you are clenching your teeth, allow your lower jaw to relax so that your teeth slightly separate. Soften your throat. Focus on your chest and visualize your heart opening and your chest expanding so that you experience the sensations of lightness and being free. Let the feeling of lightness infiltrate your abdomen and pelvis. Notice if you are tensing the muscles in your pelvis floor and if so, let go. Allow your palms to soften and observe how your fingers lightly curl as you relax. Stay with and embrace these sensations.

3 Spend a few minutes in silence in full awareness of your breath and of the subtle sensations and changes in your body as you let go and allow yourself to be completely at ease.

THE FINAL RELEASE

Do not come out of your relaxation suddenly. Take your time, releasing carefully and attentively. If you are in corpse pose, gently roll your head from side to side for several repetitions. Now bend your knees and squeeze them in towards your chest. Roll on your back, clockwise, anticlockwise, side to side and back and forth. Enjoy the massaging effect on your back and spine. Finally roll onto your right side, taking your right arm behind you and raising your knee. Stay on your side for a few moments until you are ready to come up, then ease yourself to sitting.

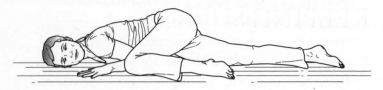

Conclusion

If you are already fairly supple, look no further than yoga for the ultimate form of exercise to keep you that way. It's wonderfully calming, too, as the centuries-old moves and postures have been carefully designed to promote spiritual awareness and tranquil contemplation. However, treat yoga with respect … It is not for every older person, as it can be deceptively demanding and will really test your bones, joints and muscles in many postures. If you are worried that something might go "twang" as you attempt one of the positions described above, do consult your doctor before you begin. Having said that, the more you practise this wonderful discipline, the more your body will feel less like old piano legs and more like banjo strings!

Chapter 7

OTHER EXERCISES FOR KEEPING SUPPLE

If, after reading through this book and considering the many different forms of exercise on offer, you still can't find something that suits you, then try some of the other exercises covered in this chapter. If suppleness is your goal, then you could do a lot worse than these. Whereas a number of the sports and exercises dealt with in this book will help you build general fitness and strength as well as flexibility, the following exercises are devoted primarily to promoting pure suppleness.

With these exercises, there is no fancy equipment involved, no daft clothing, and you won't have to go further than your bedroom floor to perform them. So, clear a space – and enjoy!

The Benefits of "Core Stability"

We begin with the wonderfully-named "core stability".
Now, you might think this sounds like something to do with
protons and questionable nuclear energy, but core stability
is actually the effective use of the core muscles to help
stabilize the spine, allowing your limbs to move more freely.

Good core stability means you can keep your mid-
section rigid without forces such as gravity affecting
your movements. If your mid-section is currently very
wobbly, then these are the exercises for you! The positive
effects of core stability include reducing the likelihood
of injury, better posture, increased agility and flexibility
and improved coordination. Yes, we can make a younger-
feeling man or woman of you yet! Core training also
helps to improve your "proprioception" – the way your
body reacts and recovers from being unbalanced. This can
be very useful indeed as you increasingly encounter the
general wooziness and wobbliness which is sadly often
associated with advancing years.

Core training aims to increase your core stability by
developing trunk fitness, which is relevant to everyday life
rather than just to sport. These days you might not find
yourself in a situation where you need to do 100 sit-ups
very often, but when you are reaching down to pick up the
dog or one of the grandchildren, for example, you require
a fundamental core strength in order not only to pick up
the object but also to avoid injuring yourself.

Beyond the basic exercises that we offer here, there are many other ways of improving core stability, from traditional abdominal exercises to movement therapies such as pilates and yoga (see Chapter 6) and even water-based exercise (see Chapter 4). If you're interested in this particular aspect of exercising, why not give these a try as well? However you decide to strengthen your core, to really capture the benefits of core strength – including better alignment, balance and functional movement (as well as a flat tummy) – it is necessary to work the deep, underlying abdominal and back musculature.

How to train your core

Traditional abdominal muscle training can be boring for many people, and as you get older, what people think of your "abs" is probably neither here nor there. After all, your days of posing on the beach and at the poolside are probably over – let's leave that to the youngsters!

Endless stomach "crunches" (see page 131) are not only monotonous, but also ineffective because they don't target the really deep muscles. The abdominals are muscles just like any other and should be trained using the same principles as any other muscle group. They should be loaded with resistance, and challenged in a variety of ways – by lateral (side) flexion, bending forwards and backwards, and rotation. If basic strength and suppleness is the goal, hundreds of repetitions are not necessary. Core strength should be developed gradually, to decrease the risk of injury, particularly in older people. When starting out on a core training programme, you need to progress properly – and carefully:

- Start with the easiest movements and progress to more difficult movements as you get the hang of it.
- Initially, you may not require any extra load but, as you adapt, you can increase the resistance by using weights, changing your position, etc.
- Perform all movements in a slow and controlled manner until coordination, strength and confidence permit higher-speed movements.
- To increase the complexity and muscle demands of the exercises, many moves can be performed lying prone (face down) or supine (on your back) on an exercise ball or another unstable platform, once you have mastered them on the floor.

Three Exercises for Improved Core Stability

Here are three of the best trunk-tightening and core-strengthening exercises for people of a certain age. They are not too difficult, but stop if you feel any pain!

ROLL DOWN THE WALL

This is a great warm-up exercise for your back. The aim is to lengthen the spine and increase its flexibility, strengthen your abdominal muscles and help build core strength. Keep your breathing controlled and regular throughout.

1 Stand about 30cm (1ft) away from a wall with your feet parallel and hip-width apart, and your knees slightly bent. Lean back on the wall to support your spine. Put your spine in neutral (see page 34) and tighten your abdominal muscles.

2 Slowly roll down off the wall by dropping your chin towards your chest and letting the weight of your head draw you downwards, trying to avoid swaying from side to side. Let your arms dangle down.

3 Roll down as far as is comfortable (ideally, until your hands touch the floor) then reverse the motion so that you come back up to a standing position.

4 Perform five repetitions.

STANDING FORWARD BEND

This exercise stretches and strengthens your spine, helps you to stand properly and helps build core strength.

1 Stand up straight with your spine in neutral (normal position) and your feet close together, knees slightly bent and your arms by your side. Set your abdominal muscles.

2 Bend forwards until your body is at a 90-degree angle and your hands are behind you.

3 Return to the start position.

4 Perform five repetitions.

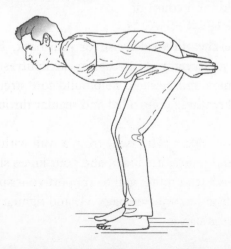

CAUTION

Both the exercises described above involve forward flexion (bending) of the spine, and you should consult your doctor before doing them if you have a history of lower-back problems.

SIDE STANDING LEG LIFT

This works your abdominal muscles and back extensors as well as your quadriceps, hamstrings and gluteals (buttock muscles).

1 Stand up straight with your spine in neutral, your feet hip-width apart and arms by your sides. Set your abdominal muscles.
2 Support your body weight on your right leg and lift your left leg to the side. As you do this extend your right arm forwards and your left arm out to the side. Hold for a count of three.
3 Repeat on the other side.
4 Perform six to eight repetitions.

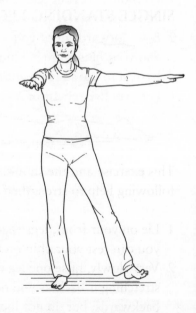

Tip
If you want to really push yourself, add ankle weights for an increased challenge – but only when you can perform the leg lifts perfectly.

Three Exercises for a Stronger, More Supple Back

Back problems are common among older people (and many younger ones too). It's no surprise when you think about it – your back has done an awful lot of work over the years!
Consequently, the more you can do to strengthen your back and make it more supple, the better.

SINGLE STANDING LEG LIFT

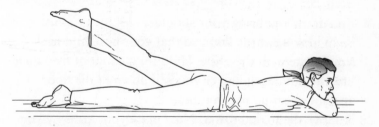

This exercise and the shoulder raise and double leg lift following help to strengthen the muscles of the back.

1 Lie on your front, legs together and arms folded so that you can rest your chin on them.
2 Very slowly, raise one leg as you breathe in. Keep stretching it back as you do so, with the toes pointing backwards, but do not lock your knee. Lift the leg as far as you can without feeling strain in the back, then hold

for a count of five, breathing normally. Bring the leg
back down to the floor as you breathe out, and repeat
up to ten times.
3 Do the same with the other leg, again lifting it only as
far as feels comfortable. It doesn't matter if one leg lifts
up higher than the other as long as it is comfortable.

SHOULD RAISE AND DOUBLE LEG LIFT

The shoulder raise and double leg lifts are more difficult
than the previous exercise, so you should only try them if
you can do single leg lifts easily.

1 Lie on your front, legs together, as in the single leg lifts,
and rest your head on a towel. This time bring your
hands behind your back, placing the back of your left
hand in the palm of your right, and rest them on your
buttocks.
2 Breathe in and bring your shoulders off the ground.
Keep looking at the floor, so that your head and neck
stay in line with the spine. Hold for a count of five, then
breathe out as you lower yourself down to the floor
again. Repeat up to ten times.
3 Remove the folded towel. Now place your arms by your
sides, palms facing upwards. Turn your head to one side
so that you rest your face on the mat. Then breathe in
and raise both legs off the floor simultaneously. Hold for
a count of five, then breathe out and return to the floor.
Repeat up to ten times.

MOY COMPLEX

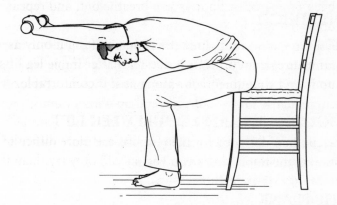

This exercise is also known as the "row, rotate and press" and is a great way to tone the muscles in your back, without having to use the complicated machinery that you would find in a gym.

1 Sit on the edge of a chair with a dumbbell or a can of soup in each hand.
2 Bend over from the waist so that your chest is resting on your knees. Make sure your head and neck are relaxed, so that you're looking down towards the floor.
3 Start with your hands resting on the floor, with elbows slightly bent, then bend your arms and bring your hands up to shoulder level.
4 Rotate your wrists and extend your arms out in front of you so that they're parallel to the floor.
5 Retrace your steps so you're back in the step 2 position, then repeat the movement.

Three Exercises for a Toned, Flat Stomach

These exercises will tighten the abdominal muscles without putting any strain on your back. They're a simple way to tone and strengthen your abdominal muscles. Perform them regularly and you'll soon end up with a tummy like the one you had 20 years ago! Always use a proper exercise mat designed for the purpose and clear plenty of space on the floor before you begin.

THE PLANK

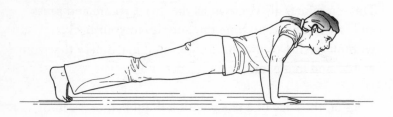

This doesn't sound or look too taxing but, if you do it right, you'll find that it's one of the most intense exercises in this whole book, and very effective for toning the abdominal muscles. Let's hope you don't feel like you have walked the plank afterwards ...!

1 Lie on the floor on your front, resting your forehead on the backs of your hands.
2 Keeping your elbows bent, slide your hands across the floor, rotating from the shoulders, until you find your perfect "push-up" position at either side of your chest.

3 Curl your toes underneath you and push up off the floor with your hands. Keep your elbows soft to stop them locking, and keep your neck and head relaxed and in line with your spine.

4 Hold the pose for ten seconds, then gently lower yourself back down to the floor again. Remember to breathe during the exercise.

CRUNCHES

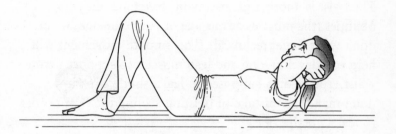

Unfortunately we are not talking about the golden chocolate treat from the newsagent, but rather an intense workout for your stomach muscles, and a great way of getting a washboard-flat tummy – should you desire such a thing.

1 Lie on the floor, with your knees bent and feet (apart) flat on the floor in line with your hips. Make sure your lower back is pressed into the floor. Put your hands behind your head to support your neck.

2 Engage your stomach muscles, by pulling your abdominals toward your spine, and lift your upper body off the floor as far as you can without arching

your lower back. You may find that you can't get up very high, but it's the effort of moving that counts, so make sure that you're pushing yourself as hard as you comfortably can. With practice, you may be able to sit up completely.

3 When you can't go any further, pause for one second. Then gently lower yourself back down into the starting position and repeat.

TWIST

The twist is another great way of stretching out your obliques (the muscles at the side of your stomach, if you don't want to get technical). This smooth movement will help you develop long and lean muscles to support a trim waist. You're only supposed to feel a subtle stretch, so don't make the mistake of twisting around too far in order to feel a greater one.

1 Stand with feet hip-width apart. Your feet should be flat on the floor and toes should be facing forwards.
2 Extend both arms out to the sides, at shoulder height.
3 Keeping your arms straight, gently rotate from the hip around to the left. Your hips and pelvis should remain facing forwards.
4 Hold the position for two sets of seven seconds, until you feel the stretch in your waist. Slowly return to the starting position and then repeat on your right side.

Three Exercises for Toned and Flexible Legs

When it comes to suppleness, do you feel that your legs in particular have stiffened up as you have got older? Well, this should be no surprise as it is particularly common for the thighs to tighten up, which can cause the hips and pelvis to rotate backwards, resulting in bad posture. However, this problem can be effectively countered with these stretches.

SEATED HAMSTRING STRETCH

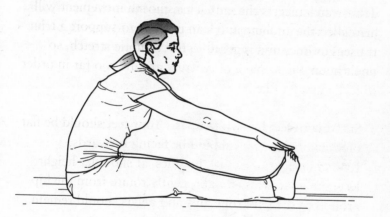

The hamstrings are the muscles running up the backs of the thighs to your bottom. It is common for older people to suffer with tight hamstrings, especially if they don't do enough exercise or, contrarily, if they do a lot of sport, which is why it's great to stretch them out. This stretch works both hamstrings at the same time, so you get double the benefit!

1 Sit down on the floor with your legs straight out in front of you, keeping your feet flexed. Sit up straight so that your back is not hunched and place your hands firmly on your hips.

2 Lean forward from the hips, letting your upper body drop down towards your feet. You can extend your arms and try to touch your toes, although if you do this, make sure that you don't curve your back.

3 Hold for ten seconds but don't bounce. Return to the starting position and repeat twice more.

INNER THIGH STRETCH

This stretch targets the muscles in the inner thighs, which are called the adductors. It's an easy way to stretch both the legs at once and is great if you combine it with a short meditation.

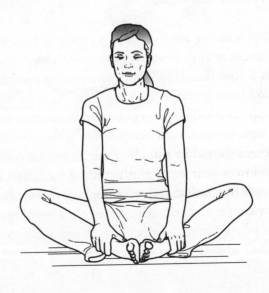

1 Sit on the floor with knees bent and soles of your feet pressed together so you're in a "frog" position. Hold the soles of your feet together with both hands.
2 Sit up, so your back is straight, and pull your tummy muscles in towards your spine.
3 Using the muscles in your inner thighs, push your knees down towards the floor. Make sure you don't bounce your knees.
4 When you've got your knees as far down as they can go, hold the stretch for ten seconds. Slowly release, then hold for two more sets of ten seconds.

CALF STRETCH

If you do a lot of running or walking, you may find that your calves feel tight and inflexible. Contrarily, they might feel like this due to lack of exercise! This stretch will help them feel loose and tension-free.

1 Get down on the floor on your hands and knees, with your knees resting directly below your hips and your hands below your shoulders. Curl your toes under so they are resting on the floor.
2 Push up off the floor with both hands and straighten your legs, pushing your bottom into the air. Your elbows and knees should be soft.
3 Try to lower your heels gently to the floor. Hold for three sets of ten seconds, returning to the start position in-between.

Three Exercises for Toned and Supple Arms

There are numerous benefits to keeping your arms in good shape. If you exercise them regularly, not only will they look good, they will be powerful and efficient as well. For centuries arm strength has been associated with youth and vitality in both sexes, so why not keep yours fit and strong?

INNER ARM STRETCH
This targets all the muscles in your upper arms – you'll be surprised at how easy it is to feel the stretch.

1 Stand in an open doorframe, with your abdominals tight and body straight.
2 Hold on to the doorframe with your left hand just below shoulder level, or as high as is comfortable. Take a big step forwards so your left arm is extended out behind you. Keeping your hips facing forwards and your head and neck in line with your spine, rotate your upper body to the right until you feel the stretch in your left arm. Lean forwards to feel a greater stretch.
3 Hold for two sets of seven seconds then turn around, step forwards, and repeat the stretch with your right arm.

TRICEPS SQUEEZE BACK

This is an easy-to-perform standing exercise that will tone the back of your upper arms creating a long, toned triceps muscle and banishing any wobbly arms. The other great thing with this exercise is that it also stretches your chest muscles, which helps promote good posture.

1 Stand with good posture and your knees slightly bent. Hold the weights keeping your arms by your side, with your palms facing away from you backwards.

2 Lift your chest and pull your shoulders back.

3 Lift both arms directly behind you, and feel this working through your triceps. Hold your arms at the highest point, then slowly lower back to the start position.

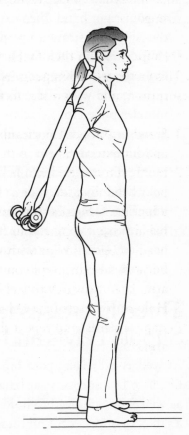

TRICEPS PONY TAIL

This standing triceps exercise
is one of the best ways to tone
flabby upper arms.

1 Stand with good posture. Bend
   your knees slightly and pull in
   your stomach. Place a weight
   in your right hand, then extend
   the right arm straight up and
   support it with the other arm
   from the front. Keep a good
   posture and your abdominal
   muscles pulled in.
2 Now simply bend at the elbow
   of your extended arm so that
   the weight comes down behind
   your head towards your
   upper back. Slowly straighten
   the arm back up to the start
   position. Do all your repetitions on
   one arm and then repeat on the other arm.

Three Exercises for a Supple Pelvis and Hips

As well as exercising your hip and thigh muscles, these leg
lifts help to improve your balance and exercise your pelvis
as well. You will need to hold on to the back of a chair or
a table for support for all these exercises. Keep all your
movements smooth and fluid and move only as far as is
comfortable for your body.

LATERAL LEG RAISE

This exercise helps to tone
and tighten your outer
thigh muscles and your
hips, as well as improve
your balance.

1 Stand up straight with
  good posture, hands
  by your sides, and feet
  together, holding on to
  the back of a chair with
  both hands for balance.
2 Tighten your abdominal
  muscles by gently
  drawing in your navel towards your spine (which will
  protect your lower back muscles).
3 Simply raise one leg out to the side about 45 degrees.
  Keep your toes pointing forwards and hold for a count
  of three. Relax and do all your repetitions on one leg
  then repeat using the other leg.

FRONT LEG RAISE

This exercise strengthens and tones the front of your
thighs (quadriceps) and increases your hip flexibility. It
also helps with balance.

1 Stand up straight with your feet together and hold on
  to the back of a chair sideways with your left hand to
  balance. Tighten your stomach muscles.
2 With your left leg slightly bent, raise your right leg out
  in front of you as far as is comfortable.

3 Hold for a count of three.
4 Lower and do all your repetitions on one leg then repeat
   on the other leg.

REAR LEG RAISE

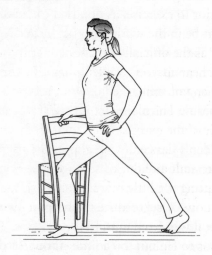

This strengthens and tones the buttocks, lower back, back
of hips and hamstrings. It also helps with your balance.
For best results, keep your buttocks tensed throughout –
it's harder but better for you in the long run!

1 Stand up straight with your feet together and use your
   right hand to hold on to the back of a chair sideways to
   help you balance.
2 Pull in your stomach muscles to support your back and
   tighten your buttock muscles.
3 Take your left leg back, and touch the floor with your
   toes. Hold this position for a count of three then return
   to the start. Do all your repetitions on one leg then
   repeat on the other leg.

Warming Down

After any form of exercise, it is advisable to "warm down" for a little while before stopping completely. This is basically the same as "cooling down", but presumably because you "warm up" prior to exercise, as opposed to "cooling up", the powers that be in the world of sport have deemed that "warm down" is the officially sanctioned term for quietly collapsing in a heap as you wonder what on earth you were thinking of when you embarked on your series of exercises sometime earlier ... The plain fact is that you might feel tired as a result of the exercises, but your body won't thank you if you suddenly cease moving altogether after what might have been half an hour or so of relatively vigorous activity. So, putting it a little more technically, the purpose of the "warm down" is to reduce the heart rate and help to remove fluid build-up from around the muscles. The best way to do this is to embark on a little static stretching, not dissimilar to what you were doing when you were warming up. For example, a hamstring stretch will probably help your legs feel less wobbly and a good, slow back extension while lying on your front will cool down those muscles and reduce soreness later on.

Stand up straight and slowly pull your foot up behind you, and you are performing a quadriceps stretch. Although this sounds fancy and highly technical, it's actually terribly simple and will gently ease the muscles at the front of your thighs.

Kneel on the floor and push your arm down your back as far as it will go while remaining in line with your head, and you will give your triceps a good old stretch.

Finally, if you can face it, lie on your back and draw
your knees up towards your chest. Now gently cross
one leg over the other, one at a time. If this warm-down
exercise doesn't tie you in knots, it will give your gluteals
a soothing treat that will dissipate any nasty lactic acid
that might still be hanging around, likely to cause you pain
later on.

Take your time and let your heart rate drop steadily. Then,
reach for the teapot – or better still, have your other half
make a cup for you.

Conclusion

Well, there you are ... If you don't feel more supple by
now, then there is not a lot more we can do! Seriously
though, if you have followed the instructions in this
chapter carefully, hopefully your body will now be
feeling the benefits of the stretches featured above. Try
an experiment: reach down and touch your toes. Did you
manage it? Was it easier than it would have been a few
weeks ago? If the answer is yes, you are well on the way to
achieving a more supple body.

Chapter 8

DIET FOR SUPPLENESS

Believe it or not, the way you eat will have a significant effect on how supple your bones, joints and muscles are as you venture through the happy vale of wrinklydom. If you have spent your life indulging yourself with pies, burgers and chips, too much booze and lots of cakes and sweets, the chances are that you are (a) not quite as slim as you should or might like to be, and (b) struggling somewhat with the extra weight and general bodily fallout that such a diet will engender over a period of years. The actor Marlon Brando comes to mind. Once a paragon of male perfection with, to many people's eyes, the ideal looks and physique, by the time he made the classic Vietnam war film *Apocalypse Now* in 1979 he was a grotesque, enormous parody of himself, forced to hide in the shadows and shave his head in a vain attempt to look slimmer, after years of scoffing down vast quantities of junk food.

An extreme example perhaps – but if you are uneasily stroking your belly as you read this and wondering if you too could ever have "been a contender", maybe you haven't been paying your own diet enough attention? However, however ... As with a surprising number of things in the world of advancing years, the good news is that it is never too late to change. You can lose weight, turn back the tide of calories, resist sweet temptation and become slimmer and more supple into the bargain. It's just a case of finding the right food swaps – because there are a surprising number of tasty morsels out there in the seemingly colourless world of "sensible eating" that are in fact remarkably good for you. Read on ...

The Importance of Eating Well

Eating well is important throughout life and is central to remaining healthy and feeling youthful as you get older. The key is a balanced diet made up of foods that provide plenty of energy and satisfaction without overloading or damaging your body. This chapter offers tips on the best foods to eat, what to avoid and how to control and monitor your diet, while still enjoying your life. We don't expect you to go to nutritional boot camp; we just want to help you find a few ways to improve your diet and take some of the pressure off your knee and hip joints, along with your heart, liver, lungs – the list is endless!

"You are what you eat", or so the old saying goes. As scientific research reveals more and more about our bodies and the nutritional value of foods, there would appear to be a great deal of truth in this statement. One thing is for sure: what you eat will have a great bearing on how young you look and feel.

Eating for Youthfulness

You eat primarily to stay alive, but making conscious choices about what you eat and how you eat it can have a hugely beneficial effect on your health and appearance as well as simply sustaining you. It is mainly nutrition, not the fact of ageing itself, that determines the body's internal chemistry, and that chemistry determines, in large part, the quality and resilience of virtually every organ, cell and system in the body. Consequently, everything from the condition of your skin to the quality of your bones, brain and connective tissue is determined in part by what you eat. As a result, your eating habits are a major determinant in how quickly you begin to see and feel the effects of ageing – and how fast you stiffen up accordingly. Naturally, then, the better you eat the better you will look and feel – and the more lithely you will move!

Eating Realistically

While this chapter is full of great advice about what and how to eat in order to stay feeling young and supple, we acknowledge that you are only human (if somewhat wrinkly) and that consequently it is not always easy to stick to a balanced, healthy diet – the straight and narrow of eating. However, if you observe these basic rules on top of the detailed advice in the following pages, you won't go far wrong:

- Avoid transfats, found in fast foods and products advertising hydrogenated oils – these cause internal inflammation, lead to the body's inability to regenerate organs and will shorten your longevity.
- Avoid too much sugar – the body is unable to break down large amounts of sugar and in the process makes you look older by creating (more) wrinkles.
- Avoid carbohydrate overload – similar to sugar, excess carbohydrates stress the body. This can age the body by leading to type 2 diabetes, metabolic syndrome and heart disease.
- Avoid waiting to eat until you are starving – the hormone ghrelin is released when your brain senses it's hungry. It can take 30 minutes to normalize your ghrelin levels. This can trigger overeating and lead to obesity.
- Avoid eating when stressed – cortisol, a stress hormone, can prevent digestion, impact the stomach's acidity levels preventing nutrient absorption and make you more apt to make unhealthy food choices and overeat.

Balance Your Diet

A diet based on starchy foods such as rice and pasta, with plenty of fruit and vegetables, some protein-rich foods like meat, fish and lentils, and some milk and dairy foods (as well as not too much fat, salt or sugar) will give you all the nutrients that you need to stay young and supple longer. Put the digestives away and go easy on that single malt – it's time to put balance back in your diet and a spring back in your step. Sorry if that sounds boring, but don't worry, there's some good stuff coming up in a little while ...

Balance for good health

As with so many things in life – as a wise person such as yourself will know – when it comes to a healthy diet, balance is the key to getting it right. This means eating a wide variety of foods in the right proportions. However, in our hectic modern lives, achieving that balance can sometimes be difficult. At the end of a long day, it can be tempting to grab the first ready meal that comes to hand on the supermarket shelf. It is fine to do this occasionally, but many ready meals contain high levels of fat, added sugar and salt. If you consume ready meals too often, at the expense of fresh whole foods, they will upset the balance in your diet, will pile on the pounds and will hasten that gradual process of bodily stagnation and congealing that you simply must avoid in order to remain supple.

The five key food groups

All the food we eat can be divided into five groups. For a healthy diet, you need to eat the right balance of these groups:

- Fruit and vegetables.
- Starchy foods, such as rice, pasta, bread and potatoes. Choose wholegrain varieties whenever you can.
- Meat, fish, eggs and beans.
- Milk and dairy foods.
- Foods containing fat and sugar.

Many people eat too much fat, sugar and salt, and not enough fruit, vegetables and fibre.

Fibre from fruit and vegetables

Fruit and vegetables are a vital source of vitamins and minerals. Ideally, you should eat at least five portions of a variety of fruit and vegetables every day. In fact, these days the health police are even recommending seven! (Can you imagine forcing down seven individual portions of fruit and veg every day? Anyone would think you were the man from Del Monte!) However, there is some fairly persuasive evidence that people who eat at least five portions a day are at lower risk of heart disease, stroke and some cancers. And once again, this applies throughout life, whatever your vintage ...

Energy from starch

Starchy foods such as bread, cereals, potatoes, pasta and maize are an important part of a healthy diet. They are a good source of energy and the main source of a range of nutrients in our diet. Starchy foods are fuel for your body. Starchy foods should make up around one third of everything you eat. So, if you have loved potatoes all your days, the good news is that you can keep 'em coming!

Protein from meat, fish, eggs and beans

These foods are all good sources of protein, which is essential for growth and repair of the body. They are also good sources of a range of vitamins and minerals. Around 15 per cent of the calories that we eat each day should come from protein. Watch out for beans, though – they can have unfortunate side effects, particularly on the older digestive tract – and don't eat too many eggs or too much red meat. Variety is the key!

Milk and dairy foods for calcium and protein

Cheese and yogurt are good sources of protein, but do your heart a favour and stick to brie rather than roquefort. A reasonable rule of thumb with cheese is that the stronger it smells and the greasier it looks, the more it will clog up your arteries. Blue veins are a bit of a give away, too. Stilton and gorgonzola might be lovely, but they probably won't aid your quest to become super supple.

All these foods also contain calcium, which helps to keep your bones healthy and strong. However, as alluded to above, some dairy products are high in saturated fat, which can raise blood cholesterol levels and will increase the risk of heart disease.

Fat and sugar in moderation

Many people eat too much fat and too much sugar, and this is one of the fastest ways to accelerate the ageing process. Fats and sugar are both good sources of energy for the body, but if you eat too much of them you will consume more energy than you burn. This generally means that you will put on weight. This can lead to obesity, which will increase your risk of type 2 diabetes, heart disease and certain cancers. The extra weight will also put pressure on your joints – especially those of your knees and hips – which could affect your general suppleness and mobility. There is no need to avoid fat and sugars altogether – and doubtless your afternoons out with friends would never be the same again if you did! – but once again moderation is the watchword.

Eat Superfoods for Super Health and Suppleness

Superfoods are rich in phytochemicals that can ward off such modern-day ills as heart disease, cancer and osteoporosis. Eat these powerful foods often for incredible health and fitness benefits and to keep you looking and feeling as young and bouncy as possible.

TOP TEN SUPERFOODS

1 SOY Soy products contain all the amino acids required to create a complete protein, making them ideal substitutes for meat and fish. No longer frowned upon as "poor man's meat"!

2 COLLARD GREENS Dark green leafy vegetables, like broccoli, are a rich source of the nutrients that suppress the growth of cancer cells. They sound off-putting, but are actually jolly tasty.

3 GARLIC Along with its cousins the shallot, onion and leek, garlic has many benefits. It boosts immune function and regulates cholesterol and blood pressure levels to prevent heart disease and stroke. It does make your breath smell, though ...

4 WHEATGRASS JUICE As a potent detoxifier and antibacterial agent, wheatgrass clears poisons from the body and enhances immune and liver function. Don't be put off by the hippy-ish connotations.

---

5 SHIITAKE MUSHROOM Terrible name, great effects. Shiitake mushrooms are valued as powerful cancer fighters. They help fight disease by stimulating the immune system.

6 FLAXSEED OIL This is a beneficial omega-3 essential fatty acid (EFA) – essential for optimal brain and cell function, but also the building block for the hormones that regulate your body's inflammation systems. Good stuff!

7 GREEN TEA Low in caffeine and high in catechins, green tea is one of the best anti-tumour foods. Studies have shown that drinking green tea daily for at least six months reduces the chances of contracting cancer. Nicer than grass …

8 SEAWEED This family of sea vegetables is extremely high in antioxidants, fibre, magnesium, potassium and iron. Seaweed also contains many anti-inflammatory, immune-boosting and tumour-suppressing constituents. Ahoy there!

9 BLACKCURRANTS Although we usually think of citrus fruits as the main source of vitamin C, blackcurrants actually contain much more of this vital nutrient.

10 ALMONDS These tasty nuts have tremendous health potential. They are high in fat – but it's the "good" fat. They are also packed with vitamins and minerals. And they make very nice liqueurs (for special occasions).

Take Vitamins for Improved Strength and Vitality

Vitamins are essential substances that cannot be manufactured by the body. We all need small amounts of vitamins for growth and development and in order to stay healthy and live a long life. Without vitamins the body simply cannot survive. Take them daily as supplements to your diet.

What are vitamins?

The term vitamin is derived from the phrase "vital amine". There are two types.

- Fat-soluble vitamins (A, D, E and K) are usually found in meat and meat products, animal fat and vegetable oils, dairy products and fish. They are transported around the body in fat, and your body stores any excess in the liver and fatty tissues. This means that you do not need to get them from food sources every day.

- Water-soluble vitamins (B, C, folic acid) are found in meat, fish, fruit, vegetables and wholegrains. They are transported around the body in water. This means your body cannot store them because you pass the excess through urine. You need to eat foods containing these vitamins every day. Water-soluble vitamins can be destroyed by cooking, so steam and grill foods rather than boiling them.

Ensuring you get what you need

We all need vitamins to live a long and healthy life, and a varied diet is essential if we are to obtain the nutrients we need. Plenty of foods naturally contain vitamins, and some popular foods such as breakfast cereals are fortified with vitamins and minerals. If for any reason you are unable to get all the vitamins that you need from your daily diet – perhaps due to being too busy, or in a strange environment – then it is important to supplement your meals with ready-prepared tablets and liquids that are widely available from health shops and supermarkets.

Don't take too many!

Too little of just one vitamin may disturb your body's balance and cause health problems, but taking too many vitamins can also be dangerous. This is especially true of the fat-soluble vitamins A, D, E and K, because it is harder for the body to get rid of any excess through urine.

THE BEST FOODS FOR HEALTHY JOINTS

1 WILD SALMON Salmon is a great source of one of
nature's best anti-inflammatory compounds: omega-3
fatty acids. Choose wild salmon – farmed varieties have
fewer omega-3s and sometimes none at all. Canned
salmon typically comes from wild fish, so it's a good
low-cost option. Sockeye salmon also contains vitamin
D, essential for healthy joints and bones.

2 ALMONDS Almonds are one of the best vitamin
E sources, which protects the outer membrane of
joint cells. This makes it a first-line defender against
free radicals. If you're not a fan of these nuts, munch
on sunflower seeds or peanuts instead. Both are rich
in E.

3 PAPAYA People who consumed the lowest amounts
of vitamin C were three times more likely to develop
rheumatoid arthritis than those who consumed more,
according to a 2004 study published in the Annals of
Rheumatic Diseases. This antioxidant penetrates into
cells, where it protects DNA from free-radical damage.
Guess what? Which fruit has the most vitamin C? It's not
oranges. Papayas have almost twice as much C, plus a
hefty dose of beta-carotene, another good antioxidant for
joint health.

4 APPLES Collagen, the fibrous protein that keeps
skin firm and wrinkle-free, is the main component of
cartilage and acts like a shock absorber in your joints,
helping them withstand years of pounding and

pressure. Collagen breakdown is often a critical step in osteoarthritis development. An apple a day can help keep arthritis at bay. It's rich in quercetin, an antioxidant that's important in building collagen and slowing its deterioration. A true friend of older folks!

5   BLACK BEANS Remember amino acids, the "building blocks" of life? They're essential for forming cartilage and every other bodily tissue. Your body naturally produces some amino acids, but you need to get others from food, namely protein. Chinese takeaways often feature black beans, but unfortunately these meals aren't very good for you!

Beans of all sorts – kidney, white, red, black – pack a protein punch: one cup has about the same amount as a pint of milk. However, black ones have an edge over the others when it comes to other joint-boosting compounds. They're richer in antioxidants, especially free-radical fighters called anthocyanins, which inhibit production of COX-2, an enzyme responsible for inflammation. They're also loaded with manganese, an indispensable mineral for healthy joints.

6   KALE When the ends of bones are brittle and frayed, the joint connecting them suffers, too. Enter calcium, the go-to mineral for healthy bones. Most of us think of milk and other dairy products as the way to get calcium. But kale is loaded with the mineral too. Want some more kale benefits? It's cholesterol-free; much lower in fat and calories than dairy; rich in joint-

protecting vitamins A, C and K; and packed with
two minerals that joints need to stay robust: copper,
which helps build collagen and ligaments, the tissue
strands that connect two bones, and manganese, which
activates enzymes needed for tissue growth and repair.

7   BROCCOLI A cousin of kale in the brassica family,
    broccoli is a winner for sulforaphane. This chemical
    may reinvigorate the body's defences against free
    radicals. Those defences decline as you age, raising the
    risk of osteoarthritis and other joint problems. Broccoli
    also has the alphabet soup of vitamins that keep joints
    well nourished – A, several Bs, C, a little E and K – not
    to mention lots of calcium and some protein.

8   GINGER Best known as a stomach soother, ginger
    has been used in Asia for centuries to reduce joint
    pain and swelling. Thanks in large part to compounds
    called gingerols, the spice has much the same effect as
    non-steroidal anti-inflammatory drugs: it clamps down
    on the production of COX-2, a key enzyme in joint
    inflammation.

THE BEST FOODS FOR MAINTAINING STRONG, SUPPLE MUSCLES

1 WHOLE EGGS A cheap and rich source of protein: 7g per egg. The yolk contains most nutrients: half the protein, vitamins A/D/E and cholesterol to naturally increase testosterone levels. Don't worry about cholesterol in eggs – recent research shows that dietary cholesterol isn't bound to blood cholesterol.

2 FISH OIL Reduces inflammation (joints/skin), lowers body fat and increases testosterone levels. You need 9000mg EPA/DHA per day. Since you'll probably struggle to get that from eating fatty fish, consider a fish oil supplement.

3 BERRIES Strong antioxidants that also prevent cancer, heart and eye diseases. Any kind works: cranberries, raspberries, blackberries, blueberries, etc. Buy fresh or frozen berries and mix them with oatmeal for a delicious and nutritious breakfast or snack.

4 YOGURT Contains bacteria that improve your gastrointestinal health. Don't buy frozen yogurt or yogurt with added sugar and fruits at the bottom. Get plain low fat yogurt and eat it with berries and flax seeds.

5   MIXED NUTS Contain mono- and polyunsaturated
    fats, proteins, fibre, vitamin E, zinc, potassium,
    magnesium, etc. Anything works: almonds, walnuts,
    cashews, hazelnuts ... Peanut butter also works as long
    as you buy natural peanut butter without added salts
    or sugars.

6   RED MEAT Protein, vitamin B12, heme iron, zinc,
    creatine, carnosine and even omega-3 if you eat grass-fed
    beef. Eat steaks and hamburgers from top ground beef or
    sirloin.

7   BROCCOLI High in cancer-fighting phytochemicals and
    anti-estrogenic indoles. Broccoli is also high in soluble
    fibre and low calorie, helping fat loss. Eat other cruciferous
    vegetables for a change: cabbage, bok choy, cauliflower,
    kale ...

8   SPINACH One of the most alkaline of all foods,
    spinach prevents muscle and bone loss, but also cancer
    and heart diseases because of its high nutrient profile.

9   TOMATOES High in lycopene, which prevents cancer.
    The lycopene in tomato paste is four times more
    concentrated than in fresh tomatoes.

10 ORANGES Contain vitamin C to fight diseases,
    magnesium to lower blood pressure, anti-oxidant beta-
    carotenes, etc. Very good for you in lots of ways!

What to Cut and What to Keep

If you want to keep supple and generally well throughout later life, it's time to lose the following foods:

- **Tea, coffee and other caffeinated drinks**
  Caffeine is a diuretic and leads to dehydration. As a stimulant it puts your body under stress and deprives it of essential nutrients. It also prevents your body from absorbing vitamins and minerals. Maybe giving this up would be the cruellest cut of all in your daily life, but it would probably do you a fair bit of good.

- **Alcohol**
  Alcohol damages the liver, muscles and brain, and depletes your body of essential vitamins and minerals. It also makes you feel wonderful, kills pain and, for a short while at least, makes you feel as though you could do anything! A tough choice, but sadly the research says it all – you should definitely give up alcohol if you want to protect your joints and muscles and whenever you are generally detoxifying. As well as containing sugar, alcohol is broken down into a toxin in your body, and the production of harmful free radicals is increased when it is being metabolized. Sad, but true.

- **Wheat**
  Wheat bran can irritate the colon. Wheat protein (gluten) is difficult to digest, and may cause bloating, constipation and/or diarrhoea. Many people are intolerant of wheat but find they can consume other grains without problems. However, if you have coeliac disease you will need to avoid all sources of gluten permanently.

- **Convenience foods, fatty and/or fried foods and products containing sugar**
These include ready meals, biscuits, cakes and spreads. Squashes and cordials also contain sugar. Diet versions are not suitable alternatives because they contain additives. Choose fresh or dried fruits and wholefood products instead, and drink water or fruit juices. Boring, yes, but this will help with your general health.

- **Meat**
Although, as we say above, meat is good for strong bones and muscles, unfortunately it creates extra work for your digestive system and in the case of red meat contains a lot of harmful saturated fat. Confusing, isn't it? What's good for you is bad for you and vice versa, and the advice seems to change every day. Eat small quantities of good quality, organic protein instead to give your body the amino acids it needs. Eggs, oily fish (from unpolluted waters) and soya are good choices.

- **Salt and sugar**
Your body needs a great deal of fluid to metabolize foods that are high in refined sugar, so if you eat a lot of these foods your body will retain a lot of water as well. Sugar disrupts blood glucose (sugar) levels. Salt prevents fluid from being removed from the body. Funny how two things that your body actually needs all your life can also be so bad for you!

- **Cow's milk products**
Milk increases the production of mucus in the body, so it is not beneficial if you are trying to detoxify yourself

160

and get fitter. It is also thought that many people lack sufficient quantities of the enzyme lactase, which is needed to digest lactose (the main sugar in milk) and therefore cannot properly digest dairy products.

Now that we've got all the so-called "bad" stuff out of the way, here's the good stuff. Eat this little lot on a regular basis and you'll feel like Fred Astaire and Ginger Rogers on mescaline for the rest of your days:

- **Apple**
  Helps excrete heavy metals and cholesterol and is cleansing for the liver and kidneys.
- **Asparagus**
  A superb "detox" food because of its diuretic effect; helps maintain healing bacteria in the intestines.
- **Broccoli**
  Like sprouts and cabbage, increases levels of glutathione, a key antioxidant that helps the liver expel toxins.
- **Carrots**
  Packed with beta-carotene, a powerful antioxidant; antibacterial and antifungal.
- **Cranberry**
  Antioxidant-rich; destroys harmful bacteria in the kidneys, bladder and urinary tract.
- **Fennel**
  Has a strong diuretic action and helps the body eliminate fats.
- **Garlic**
  A powerful antioxidant that is also excellent at eliminating toxic micro-organisms.

- **Ginger**
  Relieves abdominal bloating, nausea and diarrhoea. helps to stimulate digestive enzymes, aiding efficient digestion.
- **Globe artichoke**
  Purifies and protects the liver and has a diuretic effect on the kidneys.
- **Lemon**
  Stimulates the release of enzymes – an essential part of the liver's detoxification process.
- **Olive oil**
  A powerful antioxidant; prevents cholesterol from being transformed into a harmful free radical.
- **Onion**
  Rich in the antioxidant quercetin, which protects against free radical damage; onion enhances the activity of healthy intestinal flora and is antiviral.
- **Parsley**
  A diuretic that helps kidneys to flush out toxins; contains phytonutrients that support the liver and is rich in antioxidants.
- **Quinoa**
  An easily digested cleansing grain that is a good source of protein, vitamins and minerals.
- **Rice**
  Brown rice in particular cleans the intestines as it passes through and prevents constipation; anti-allergenic and helps stabilize blood-sugar levels.
- **Salad leaf**
  A superb antioxidant and cleanser of the digestive tract.

- **Seaweed**
  A very strong antioxidant that helps alkalinize the blood and strengthens the digestive tract.
- **Tomato**
  A rich source of the antioxidant lycopene, thought to prevent a variety of diseases.
- **Watercress**
  This simplest of vegetables purifies the blood and expels wastes from the body.
- **Yogurt**
  Live yogurt contains probiotics that reduce intestinal inflammation and fungal infections and eliminate bad bacteria that damage the gut wall.

Diet and Arthritis

Your body needs a variety of nutrients to stay healthy, so make sure you get lots of fruit and vegetables, meat and/or fish, dairy foods, and bread, rice or pasta. This is what is meant by a balanced diet.

If you suffer from arthritis at all, there are many theories about whether what you eat affects the condition. As yet there's little scientific evidence to suggest that it does, but some doctors feel special diets are worth trying as long as they don't mean missing out on vital nutrients. If you're considering going on a special diet for your arthritis, it's important to discuss it with your doctor first.

Some people with arthritis find their condition improves when they give up certain foods. One theory is that this is because of a food allergy or food intolerance.

There are many tests for determining allergies or intolerances, but the only reliable way of identifying foods that could be making your arthritis worse is by systematically excluding them from your diet. This should be done with the knowledge of your doctor and the help of a qualified dietitian. For more on this issue that is all too relevant to many of us, see Chapter 9.

A Little Bit of What You Fancy Won't Do You Any Harm

Well, if you've read all the foregoing information in this chapter, you're probably bewildered – if not terrified – by now. While it's clear what's basically good for you and what's not, there is just so much other conflicting information to absorb and who knows how much of it is accurate? Every day your newspaper doubtless brings you little nuggets of hot-off-the-press dietary information and new "scientific findings" (but how scientific are they all really?), which probably make you wonder how on earth you lived this long in the first place. Will you live longer if you follow all this brave new foodie-world type stuff? Who knows …

When all is said and done it's probably best if you just stick to that classic old bit of advice that your mother, father, granny, aunt or local taxidermist gave you all those years ago – "everything in moderation".

This is most certainly the key – and one that has applied all your life and applies right now, not only to yourself, but to everybody else much younger and prettier than you. Keep it all in balance – don't eat too much or too little of anything – and the result will doubtless be greater suppleness, happiness and any number of other things ending in "ness" ...

Having said that, the natural corollary to the statement "all things in moderation", is – a little like "glass half-full, glass half-empty" and similar clichés – the fact that "a little of what you fancy won't do you any harm". At last, some cheering news! This means, among other things, that you can:

- Drink red wine – red wine is packed with resveratrol, an antioxidant. This works to protect your body against the effects of ageing. One or two glasses of red wine a day can help keep your body feeling young.

- Eat dark chocolate – dark chocolate made from cocoa contains a large number of antioxidants that protect your body from ageing. Eating chocolate may lower your blood pressure and cholesterol while providing an energy boost.

So, it's not all bad news by any means. And all those cups of tea you probably already consume every day won't do you any harm, either. Just try to make it green tea instead of black tea ... Without any caffeine and no milk and sugar ... Oh, and no digestive biscuits ... Only kidding!

Conclusion

So, what's it to be – "eat, drink and be merry!" or "you are what you eat"? Well, a combination of the two approaches is probably the best course to take – with the word MODERATION always firmly at the forefront of your mind. Nobody expects you to adopt a monkish habit at this stage in your life – there'll be no advocacy of hairshirts and cat o'nine tails in this happy and helpful little tome – but if you are serious about KEEPING SUPPLE, then follow as much of the advice in this chapter as you possibly can. After all, there's nothing to stop you from still having the occasional blowout ...!

Chapter 9

JOINT CARE AND GENERAL HEALTH MAINTENANCE

If you've got this far through the book, you might be feeling a little stiff by now – or at least somewhat shell-shocked, if you haven't actually tried any of the prescribed exercises yet. Is there really so much to keeping supple, to keeping fit …? Well, yes – but remember that most of it is jolly good fun once you actually get started and once your body has become accustomed to being hauled out of the armchair and dragged off somewhere else to do something better for it.

It's a reciprocal, symbiotic sort of thing, though, all this exercise … If your body is going to look after you and let you get up to all these high jinks at your advanced age, you need to look after it in return. Of course, by undertaking more exercise and becoming more fit and supple, you are doing just that – but there is more to it than pure exercise.

Joint Care

Your body is basically a machine. Okay, it's not made
of metal and doesn't feature cogs and springs, but the
analogy isn't too far-fetched, if you stop and think about
it. Let's do a quick comparison with your car, sitting on the
driveway outside. For the car's bodywork, think of your
skin and muscles; for the car's engine and gearbox, think
of your heart and other organs; for the car's petrol and
oil, think of your blood and daily nutrition; for the car's
suspension and shock absorbers, think of your bones and
joints. Get the picture? Now, how old is your car? Perhaps
it is shiny and new – smelling good, running smoothly
and completely problem-free. Well, that was probably you
about 30 years ago! Then again, maybe there is a little rust
on the bodywork. Perhaps the gear changes have become
a little jerky. Is it possible that the suspension and springs
creak a little when you climb in and out, or when the car
goes over a speed bump?

Just as your car will run less efficiently and gradually
deteriorate as it ages, sadly the exact same thing will
happen to your body. And as far as the creaking noises
mentioned at the end of our little story above go, well
that's exactly what happens to your joints with the passage
of time – they start to creak a little (sometimes even
audibly!) and, if you are really unlucky, in old age they can
become arthritic.

Putting off pain and strain

At the beginning of this book we saw that there is quite a lot you can do to prevent your joints from seizing up, your muscles losing mass and strength and your bones losing density. Here are some further useful tips for taking the best possible care of your joints and for keeping them in good shape for ongoing exercise.

TOP TIPS FOR JOINTS

- Keep to your ideal weight.
- Pace your activities throughout the day – don't tackle hard physical jobs all at once. The same goes for your exercise programme; don't cram it all into one time slot and over-stress your body.
- Think about your movements as you exercise – what causes pain and discomfort; what makes things worse?
- Wear shoes with thick soft soles, which act as shock absorbers. Get a good pair of cross-trainers before you begin any of the exercise programmes discussed in this book.
- Consider buying and using specialist equipment or modifying your home and workplace to help you avoid stressful movements that promote joint pain.

Glucosamine and other joint/bone supplements

There are theories that certain foods and dietary supplements can help keep joints young and fit and stave off the onset of arthritis. If you already have a little arthritis, these foods and supplements can also help mitigate the pain and general debilitating effects of the condition.

Some of these wonder foods and dietary aids have been tested more than others and unfortunately the medical jury is still out on whether some of them really work at all. However, there is compelling evidence that the essential fatty acids found in fish oil and plant seed oils – such as sunflower oil and evening primrose oil – may help some people with rheumatoid arthritis, when taken at a dose of 3.5g daily for fish oils and up to 6g daily for evening primrose oil. Glucosamine sulphate (but not glucosamine hydrochloride), Chondroitin, and cod liver oil can help those with osteoarthritis and delay the onset of the condition. These are all widely available from chemists, supermarkets and health stores.

Other supplements you may have read or heard about include green-lipped mussels, selenium and garlic. However, there's little scientific evidence of these having positive effects for keeping joints healthy and preventing rheumatoid arthritis and hardly any at all for positive effects on the symptoms of osteoarthritis.

Consult your doctor

You should always discuss taking any such dietary supplements with your doctor, because some of them can have a deleterious effect when combined with other medication that you might already be taking. For example, glucosamine may interfere with medications for diabetes, fish oils can affect blood clotting and so should not be taken with aspirin or warfarin, and evening primrose oil may interact with anti-inflammatory medications and also anticoagulants.

Treating painful joints

If you become injured while performing any of the exercises covered in this book, you should take a few days off to recover and visit your doctor if you are at all concerned or if things don't improve over time. You might be part of the "mustn't grumble" generation, but don't suffer in silence if your joints or muscles are complaining! It's in your interests to get over an injury as quickly as you can so that you can resume your exercise programme before you lose many of the accrued benefits.

Apart from the medication that your doctor might prescribe for you, there are a few simple ways in which you can treat your painful joints yourself:

- Warmth applied to the affected area can relieve pain and stiffness. Some people buy special heat lamps or creams that produce localized heat, but a hot-water bottle can be just as effective. However, if you use one of these, make sure it's wrapped in something so that it doesn't burn you.
- An ice pack can bring relief to hot and inflamed joints, but you should seek advice from a physiotherapist first. Never apply ice directly to the skin – it can burn!
- Stress and muscle tension can make sore or arthritic joints feel much worse. Many people find that taking a long bath, listening to soothing music or using a relaxation tape can help. A physiotherapist will be able to advise you on relaxation techniques.

Conclusion

Look after your joints and they will look after you! There's nothing worse than a decline in mobility as you get older, so don't sit and wait for things to go downhill – stay supple and keep moving. You know it makes sense!

Appendix

DAILY SUPPLENESS CHALLENGES

Fancy a fitness challenge? Try the following combinations of exercises – arranged by the days of the week – and then mix them up, trying alternative combinations on different days in subsequent weeks. Keep a note of how well you cope, with dates and times to spur you on. If you find the prescribed number of exercises or repetitions too tiring, modify the number you perform as necessary. You will be amazed at your rate of progress!

MONDAY
Full body reach-up stretch (page 31) x 10 reps
Side bends stretch (page 33) x 10 reps
Easy chest stretch (page 35) x 10 reps
Three-mile walk in 60 mins
Standing forward bend (page 125) x 10 reps
Shoulder raise and double-leg lift (page 128) x 10 reps

TUESDAY
Standing pelvic tilt stretch (page 34) x 10 reps
Shoulder stretch (page 36) x 10 reps
Upper back stretch (page 37) x 10 reps
20 lengths of your local swimming pool/60 mins
swimming, mixed strokes
Moy complex (page 129) x 10 reps
The plank (page 130) x 5 reps

WEDNESDAY
Arm stretch (page 37) x 10 reps
Marching on the spot (page 38) x 100 reps
Torso rotations (page 32) x 15 reps
Five-mile cycle ride/60 mins cycling
Crunches (page 131) x 10 reps
Twist (pag 132) x 10 reps

THURSDAY
Spinal curl (page 35) x 10 reps
Easy chest stretch (page 35) x 10 reps
Standing leg lift (page 38) x 10 reps
Three yoga poses of your choice (pages 106–117)
Seated hamstring stretch (page 133) x 10 reps
Inner thigh stretch (page 134) x 10 reps

FRIDAY

Standing forward bend (page 125) x 10 reps
Upper back stretch (page 37) x 10 reps
Shoulder stretch (page 36) x 10 reps
Three-mile walk in 60 mins
Lateral leg raise (page 139)
Rear leg raise (page 140)

SATURDAY

Three warm-up exercises of your choice (pages 34–39)
Three-mile cycle ride/30 mins cycling
Three yoga poses of your choice (pages 106–117)
Calf stretch (page 135) x 10 reps
Inner arm stretch (page 136) x 10 reps
The plank (page 130) x 5 reps

SUNDAY

Three warm-up exercises of your choice (pages 34–39)
Three yoga poses of your choice (pages 106–117)
20 lengths of your local swimming pool/60 mins
swimming, mixed strokes
Triceps pony tail (page 138) x 10 reps
Triceps squeeze back (page 137) x 10 reps
Crunches (page 131) x 10 reps

Remember to take rest days in between exercise if you
feel tired and not to overdo it! If you are in any doubt
whatsoever about your ability to cope with the daily
regimes outlined above, consult your doctor before
embarking upon them.

GLOSSARY

Activities of Daily Living (ADLs)
Physical tasks of everyday living, such as bathing, and walking up the stairs. ADLs are usually factored in to a person's basal metabolic rate, so tracking calories burned for these types of movement isn't recommended when trying to lose weight.

Aerobic exercise
Any rhythmic activity that increases the body's need for oxygen by using large muscle groups continuously for at least ten minutes. The term aerobic means "with oxygen".

Agonist muscle
A muscle that is very effective in causing a certain joint movement. Also called the prime mover. On a biceps curl, the biceps is the agonist muscle that flexes the elbow joint.

Anaerobic exercise
Short lasting, high intensity activity, where the demand for oxygen from the exercise exceeds the oxygen supply.

Angina pectoris
Chest pain due to lack of blood flow (oxygen) to the heart.

Antagonist muscle
A muscle that causes movement at a joint in a direction opposite to that of the joint's agonist (prime mover).

Beta-blockers
Type of medication that reduces heart rate. Exercisers who take beta-blockers will have a lower heart rate at rest and during exercise, so the target heart rate formula cannot be used in this case.

Body composition
Amount of fat vs lean muscle tissue in the human body.

Body Mass Index (BMI)
Measure of the relationship between height and weight; calculated by dividing weight in kilograms by height in centimeters squared.

Calisthenics
Exercising using one's own body weight which helps develop muscular tone.

Cardiorespiratory fitness
Measure of the heart's ability to pump oxygen-rich blood to the muscles. Also called cardiovascular or aerobic fitness.

Cardiovascular system
A complex system consisting of the heart and blood vessels; transports nutrients, oxygen, and enzymes throughout the body and regulates temperature, water levels of cells, and acidity levels of body components.

Circuit training
Takes the participant through a series of exercise stations (which could also include strength training), with relatively brief rest intervals between each station. The purpose is to keep the heart rate elevated near the aerobic level without dropping off. The number of stations may range from four to ten.

Concentric muscle action
Force produced while the muscle is shortening in length.

Continuous training
This is the most common type of sustained aerobic exercise for fitness improvement, slowly adding more time to the workout to increase endurance.

Cool down
Lowering of body temperature following vigorous exercise. The practice of cooling down after exercise involves slowing down your level of activity gradually.

Core
A muscle group comprised of the abdominals, lower back, obliques and hips.

Cortisol
A hormone secreted by the adrenal gland that makes stored nutrients more readily available to meet energy demands. These hormone levels increase under stress, which can stimulate your appetite, leading to weight gain or difficulty losing weight.

Cross-training
Any combination of all aerobic-training methods, characterized by a variety of intensities and modes.

Detraining Principle
This principle says that once consistent exercise stops, you will eventually lose the strength that you built up. Without overload or maintenance, muscles will weaken in two weeks or less.

Diastolic blood pressure
The pressure exerted by the blood on the vessel walls during the resting portion of the cardiac cycle, measured in millimeters of mercury. The diastolic number is the bottom of the fraction. 120/80 is an average value for normal blood pressure (80 is the diastolic number). Mild high blood pressure is considered to be between 140/90 and 160/95. High blood pressure is defined by a value greater than 160/95.

DOMS (Delayed Onset Muscle Soreness)
Muscle soreness or discomfort that appears 12–48 hours after exercise. It is most likely due to microscopic tears in the muscle tissue, and it usually requires a couple of days for the repair and rebuilding process to be completed. The muscle tissue grows back stronger, leading to increased muscle mass and strength.

Eccentric contraction
A lengthening of the muscle during its contraction; controls speed of movement caused by another force.

Ectomorph
A body shape characterized by a narrow chest, narrow shoulders and long, thin muscles.

Electrolytes
Salts (ions) found in bodily fluids. Pertaining to exercise, your body loses electrolytes (sodium, potassium) when you sweat. These electrolytes need to be replaced to keep concentrations constant in the body, which is why many sports drinks include electrolytes.

Endomorph
A body shape characterized by a round face, short neck, wide hips and heavy fat storage.

Endorphins
Opiate-like hormones that are manufactured in the body and contribute to natural feelings of well-being.

EPOC (Excess Post-Exercise Oxygen Consumption)
This explains why your breathing rate remains heavy for a few minutes after a workout. Your body needs more oxygen afterwards in order to restore the oxygen stores in the blood and tissues, and to meet the oxygen requirements of the heart rate, which is still elevated.

Fixed resistance
Strength training exercises that provide a constant amount of resistance throughout the full range of motion. Examples include free weights and resistance bands.

Flexibility
The measure of the range of motion, or the amount of movement possible, at a particular joint.

Graded Exercise Test (Incremental Exercise Test)
An exercise test involving a progressive increase in work rate over time. Often graded exercise tests are used to determine the subject's maximum oxygen consumption or lactic threshold.

Heat Cramps
Muscle cramps that occur during or following exercise in warm or hot weather.

Heat exhaustion
A heat stress illness caused by significant dehydration resulting from exercise in warm or hot conditions; frequent precursor to heat stroke.

Heat stroke
A deadly heat stress illness resulting from dehydration and overexertion in warm or hot conditions; can cause body core temperature to rise from normal to 100–105°F (38–40°C) in just a few minutes.

High-density lipoprotein (HDL)
Retrieves cholesterol from the body's cells and returns it to the liver to be metabolized.

High impact
Activities that place more stress on the bones and joints, where your limbs are actually making contact

with the ground or other surface with force. Examples include: walking, running, step aerobics and sports that involve impact, like basketball or tennis.

Hypothermia
A life-threatening condition in which heat is lost from the body faster than it is produced.

Incremental Exercise Test (Graded Exercise Test)
An exercise test involving a progressive increase in work rate over time. Often these tests are used to determine the subject's maximum oxygen consumption or lactic threshold.

Interval training
Repeated intervals of exercise interspersed with intervals of relatively light exercise. This type of training provides a means of performing large amounts of high-intensity exercise in a short period of time.

Isokinetic exercise
Exercise in which the rate of movement is constantly maintained through a specific range of motion even though maximal force is exerted.

Isometric exercise
Any activity in which the muscles exert force but do not visibly change in length. For example, pushing against a wall or carrying a bag of groceries.

Isotonic exercise
Any activity in which the muscles exert force and

change in length as they lift and lower resistance. For example, bicep curls or leg extensions.

Karvonen formula
An effective method used to calculate target heart rate. It factors resting heart rate into the equation.

Lactic acid
Once thought of as a waste substance that builds up in the muscles when they are not getting enough oxygen, leading to muscle fatigue and soreness. Now, experts believe that lactic acid is beneficial to the body, acting as a "fuel" to help people continue high-intensity exercise even when oxygen consumption is low.

Lactic threshold
The point at which the level of lactic acid in the blood suddenly increases (during exercise). This is a good indication of the highest sustainable work rate. Also known as anaerobic threshold.

Lean mass
Total weight of your muscle, bone and all other body organs. (Everything in the body besides fat.)

Low-density lipoprotein (LDL)
Transports cholesterol and triglycerides from the liver to be used in various cellular processes. Also referred to as "bad" cholesterol.

Low impact
Activities that place less stress on the bones and

joints. These are better for people with joint pain, and overweight individuals whose weight can hurt their joints. Examples include: swimming, cycling and other activities where your feet (or other body parts) aren't touching the ground with force or where you are somehow supported.

Mesomorph
A body shape characterized by a large chest, long torso, solid muscle structure and significant strength.

Moderate intensity
Activities that range from 40–60 per cent of max heart rate. These activities cause a slightly increased rate of breathing, and feel light to somewhat hard. Individuals doing activity at this intensity can easily carry on a conversation.

Muscle fibres
Individual muscle cells that are the functional components of muscles.

Muscular endurance
The ability of the muscle to perform repetitive contractions over a prolonged period of time.

Muscular strength
The ability of the muscle to generate the maximum amount of force.

Obesity
A weight disorder generally defined as an accumulation

of fat beyond that considered normal for a person based on age, sex and body type.

One-Rep Max (1RM)
The amount of weight that can be lifted or moved once, but not twice; a common measure of strength.

Opposing muscles
Muscles that work in opposition to the ones you are training. For example, the bicep is the opposing muscle to the triceps.

Osteoporosis
A disease characterized by low bone mass and deterioration of bone tissue, which increases risk of fracture.

Overload Principle
This principle says that in order to train muscles, they must work harder than they are accustomed to. This "overload" will result in increased strength as the body adapts to the stress placed upon it.

Overuse Injuries
Injuries that result from the cumulative effects of repetitive (day-after-day) stresses placed on tendons, muscles, and joints.

Physical fitness
The ability to perform regular to vigorous physical activity without great fatigue.

Pilates
Exercise programs that combine dynamic stretching with movement against resistance.

Plateau
Point in an exercise programme where no additional progress is being made (gains in strength, weight loss, increased endurance, etc). One way to break through a plateau is to change the kind of activity you are doing or something about your current activity – adding hills, increasing speed, increasing distance, etc.

PNF stretching
Proprioceptive neuromuscular facilitation (PNF) stretching is a static stretch of a muscle immediately after maximally contracting it.

Rate of perceived exertion (RPE)
Scale from 1–10 that rates how you are feeling (both physically and mentally) as it relates to exercise fatigue.

Repetition (Rep)
The number of times an exercise is repeated within a single exercise "set".

Resistance training
See "Strength training"

Resting HR
Rate at which your heart beats at rest (while sitting or being inactive). Low resting heart rates are a good measure of health and fitness.

Resting Metabolic Rate (RMR)
Number of calories expended to maintain the body during resting conditions. Also referred to as basal metabolic rate.

Set
A basic unit of a workout containing the number of times (repetitions) a specific exercise is done (e.g. do three sets of five repetitions with 45kg (100lb).

Shin splint
Generic term used to describe pain in the lower leg, either on the medial (inside) or lateral side (outside) of the shin bone.

Sit and reach test
A common fitness test that determines flexibility (of the hamstrings and lower back).

Static stretching
A low force, high-duration stretch where the muscle is held at the greatest possible length for up to 30 seconds.

Strength training (resistance training)
The process of exercising with progressively heavier resistance for the purpose of strengthening the musculoskeletal system.

Tapering
The process athletes use to reduce their training load for several days prior to competition.

Target heart rate (THR)
The recommended range is 60–85 per cent of your
maximum heart rate. It represents a pace that ensures
you are training aerobically and can reasonably be
maintained.

Variable resistance
Strength training exercises that change the amount of
resistance throughout the full range of motion.

Vigorous intensity
Activities above 60 per cent of max heart rate. These
activities cause an increased rate of breathing, sweating,
and feel somewhat hard in intensity.

Warm up
To prepare for an athletic event (whether a game or a
workout session) by exercising, stretching, or practising
for a short time beforehand.

Yoga
A variety of Indian traditions geared towards self-
discipline and the realization of unity; includes
forms of exercise widely practised in the West today
that promote balance, coordination, flexibility and
meditation.

INDEX

Index

diet and 154–6
painful 171
Jump start 64

Karvonen formula 184
Knees to chest pose 107

Lactic acid 184
Lactic threshold 184
Lateral leg raise 139
Lean mass 184
Leg lift 38–9
Leg-toning exercises 133–5
Lifestyle 15
Low impact 184–5
Lunge 63, 66
Lungs 41, 58, 77–8
Lymphatic system 24

Marching on the spot 38
Meat 146, 147, 148, 160, 163
Menstruation 105
Mental health 42, 43, 59, 77
Metabolic syndrome 146
Moderate intensity 185
Movement 12
Moy complex 129
Multi-joint exercises 85
Muscles 13, 14, 15, 17
and diet 157–8
mass 84
muscle fibres 185
toning and lengthening 23
See also Stretching
Muscular endurance 185
Muscular strength 185

Nutrition See Diet

Obesity 18, 77, 185
See also Diet
Omega-3 151
One-Rep Max (1RM) 186
Opposing muscles 186
Osteoarthritis 42, 76, 155, 156, 170
Osteoporosis 14–15, 42, 76, 186
Overload Principle 186
Overuse Injuries 186
Pelvic tilt 34

Pelvis and hip exercises 138–40
Physical fitness 186
Pilates 123, 187
The Plank 130–1
Plateau 22, 187
PNF stretching 187
Posture 12, 23, 48–50, 122
Proprioception 122, 187
Proteins 16, 146, 147, 148–9, 157

Quadriceps stretch 47, 141

Rear leg raise 140
Relaxation 23
Repetition 187
Resistance training See Strength training
Resting HR 187
Retro walking 64–5
Revolved head to knee pose 117
RMR 189
Roll down the wall 124–5
Row, rotate and press 129
RPE 187
Running 17, 76

Salt 146, 147, 160
Set 189
Shin splint 189
Shoulder raise and double leg lift 128
Shoulder stretch 36
Side bends 33
Side standing leg lift 126–7
Sideways stretching 65
Single standing leg lift 127–8
Sit and reach test 189
Sleep 29, 43
Spinal curl 35
Staff pose 113–14
Standing forward bend 125–6
Static stretching 26, 45–6, 63–7, 189

Stomach-toning exercises 130–2

Strength training 189
Stretching 17, 21–40
static See Static stretching
Sugars 146, 147, 149, 159, 160
suppleness 11–12
Sweating 77
Swimming 8–9, 17, 57–74
aqua aerobics 71–4
cooling down 69
drills 68
warming up 62–7, 69

Tapering 189
Tea 151, 159, 165
THR 189
Torso rotations 32
Transfats 146
Tree pose 109–10
Triangle pose 112–13
Triceps pony tail 138
Triceps squeeze back 137
Triceps stretch 141
Twist 132

Upper back stretch 37–8

Variable resistance 189
Vigorous intensity 189
Visualization 23, 27
Vitamins 16, 78, 151, 152–3, 154, 156, 159

Walking 8, 17, 41–56
hills 51–3
posture 48–50
upper body 50–1
warming up 44–7
weightless 64–5
Warm down 141–2
Warm up 13, 17, 22, 189
for cycling 81–6
for swimming 62–7
for walking 44–7
Weight training 28, 84–8
Wheat 159
Wholegrains 16, 147
Wobble board 28

Yoga 9, 93–120, 123, 189